YOGA

The art of

Written by Elly Lloyd
With Special Thanks to Orwell Park School, Suffolk

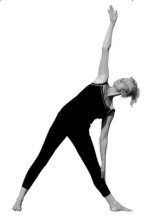

KUDOS

Published by Kudos, an imprint of Top That! Publishing plc.
Copyright © 2004 Top That! Publishing plc,
Tide Mill Way, Woodbridge, Suffolk, IP12 IAP, UK
www.kudosbooks.com
Kudos is a Trademark of Top That! Publishing plc

Contents

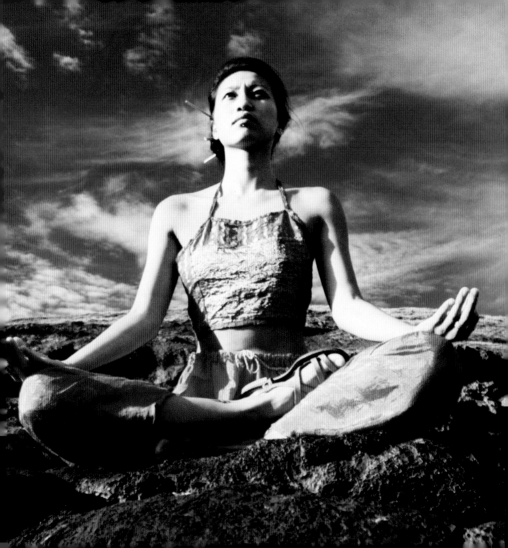

What is Yoga?

Yoga was developed in India thousands of years ago, where its techniques were kept secret and were passed down from guru to disciple by word of mouth. The word yoga is derived from the Sanskrit root 'yuj' which means to join, yoke, attach or bind. Yoga is a system of physical, mental and spiritual practices, with the ultimate goal of union between the individual self (Atman) and the higher self (Brahman). The classical yoga texts are written from a Hindu perspective and sometimes the higher self is referred to as God, but this does not mean yoga is a religion, or that certain religious beliefs must be adhered to. Yoga is a philosophy, a science and an art form.

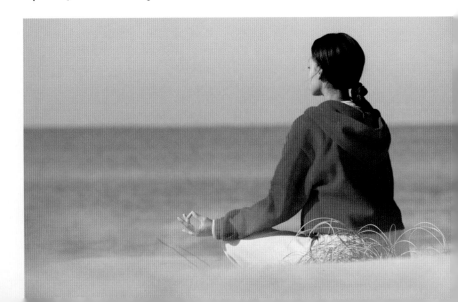

The yoga featured in this book is called Hatha yoga and is the most commonly practised form in the West and concentrates mainly on the physical body through asanas (postures) and pranayama (breathing practices). Hatha comes from the Sanskrit words 'ha' and 'tha', which mean sun and moon respectively. Hatha yoga brings about a balance between opposites – sun/moon, cool/warm, left/right, negative/positive etc. It is also a means of awakening the 'Kundalini' or universal energy, which is dormant in the base chakra (see page 114 for more detail).

Relevance of Yoga Today

Many of us are constantly under pressure, juggling family life with work and the needs each of these areas demand. All these factors build up to a stressful existence with little time being spent on the individual. Yoga is, therefore, very relevant in today's busy world.

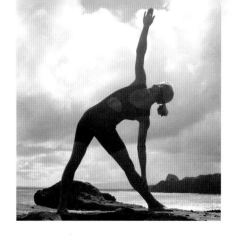

In yoga we are taught to listen to our bodies, to experience the effect the yoga practices have on us as individuals. In this way it gives us a better awareness and understanding, not only of our own needs but also those of others.

Yoga is suitable for most people, and each individual can go as deeply into it as they want. Many take it up solely for the physical aspect and this is absolutely fine. Quite often though, with regular asana practice linked with breath control, a spiritual awakening occurs.

5

Awareness of the Breath

It is very important to practise all the asanas with breath awareness. Linking respiration with the movements enhances the practice, as well as improving concentration. This is one of the reasons why yoga is much more than just physical exercise.

As a general rule, an upwards movement is done on inhalation and is used to lift out of a posture. A downwards movement is generally done on exhalation, to release tension. Exhalation is also used to relax into a posture.

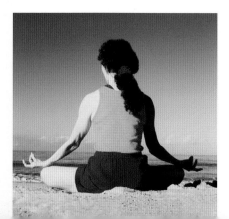

While in a posture you should try to breathe freely and not hold the breath, as this will create tension in the body and prevent relaxation into the asana.

You should breathe in and out through your nostrils, throughout all the asanas.

Listening to Your Body

Another very important thing to bear in mind is to listen to your body. Your body will tell you when it is feeling uncomfortable or under stress. In everyday life messages from the body are often ignored so that tasks can be completed – how often have you pushed yourself to do one more thing before taking a break? In yoga you should be more mindful and if a posture or movement feels 'wrong' or painful, then gently come out of it and rest for a moment.

6

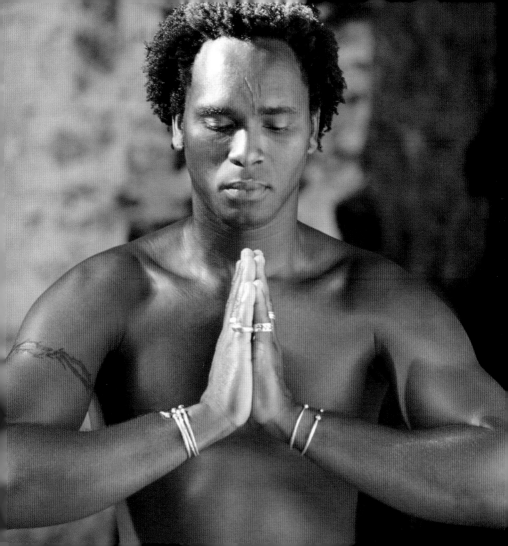

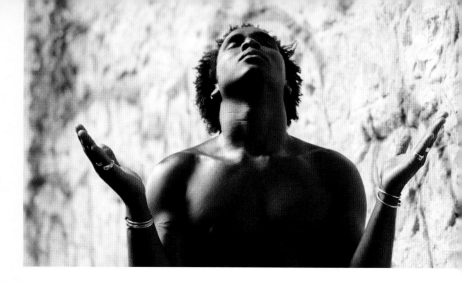

There are many benefits which can be achieved through regular yoga practice – not only for the body but for the mind as well.

Physical Benefits

The gentle stretching involved in asana practice will improve blood circulation to the cells of the body, thus enhancing muscle tone, strength and overall fitness. One should always try to hold each posture for an equal length of time on each side, so that the body becomes more balanced and symmetrical.

A well-planned programme of yoga will gently work the length of the spine, thus strengthening the muscles along it. As we get older the spaces between the vertebrae generally close up and careful stretching of the spine helps to separate the vertebrae therefore releasing pressure on the discs. Quite often backache occurs when the nerves are squeezed by the discs. Allowing them to release gently will help to reduce backache and keep the spine healthy.

In general, forward and backward bending and twisting postures massage the abdominal organs, which in turn improve digestion. As your posture

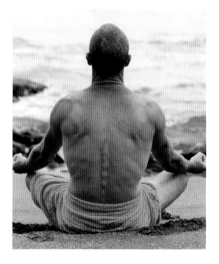

and flexibility improves you will feel more healthy, confident and rejuvenated. Better posture and a heightened awareness of the body will also improve respiration.

The main muscle responsible for breathing is the diaphragm, which has a central tendon from which muscle fibres run and attach to the spine, lower ribs and the sternum or breast bone. Movement of the spine will, therefore, affect the diaphragm and vice versa.

Inhalation occurs when the diaphragm contracts and pulls downwards. At the same time the intercostal muscles between the ribs contract, causing the ribs to move outwards and upwards. This causes a drop in air pressure within the lungs and so air is drawn into them. Exhalation happens when the muscles relax, causing the diaphragm to move up into its relaxed position and the rib cage to move inwards and downwards. This releasing of tension expels the air from the lungs. Immediately following the out breath there is a short pause before the process is repeated. Awareness of the breathe in yoga practice will reduce the breath rate, heart rate and blood pressure, all of which will lead to an improved physical wellbeing.

Mental Benefits

Merely dedicating time to yourself will be beneficial. The physical movements of yoga linked with the breath will calm the mind and improve concentration. Yoga can relieve stress, allowing more control over the emotions — especially anger. This will all add up to increased feelings of happiness and positive thinking.

Do I need to be Slim and Fit?

The answer to that question is 'no'! Your age, weight or general fitness will not stop you taking up yoga, but please ensure that you read the following section General Precautions (pages 12–21) as well as the specific precautions mentioned with each asanas before starting.

The majority of postures can be modified to suit your individual needs. If, for example, you have difficulty in getting down on to the floor and back up again, there are many postures which can be practised sitting in a chair or while standing. There are also many aids available to assist in your yoga practice; these are discussed on page 15 and will be mentioned throughout the book.

The important thing to remember is that yoga is about listening to your body, doing what feels right for you and never over-stretching. Don't be over-ambitious and expect too much of yourself. With regular practice the body will become more supple and you will gradually notice the improvement.

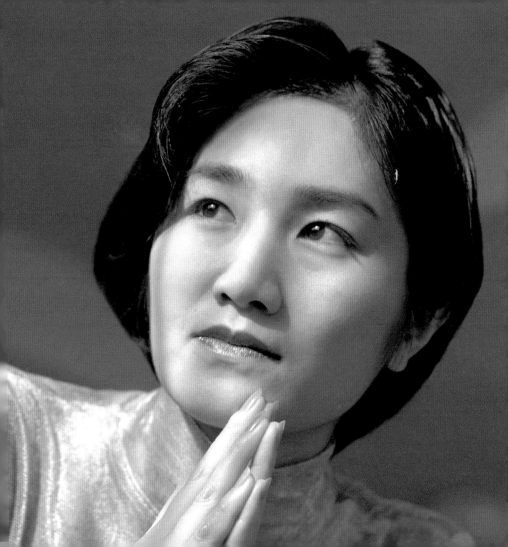

Safe Practice

Yoga is suitable for most people, but as with any new exercise regime, you should consult your doctor before starting. In particular, if you have a medical condition or have recently had surgery you must seek medical advice before taking up this holistic practice.

• Do not eat a large meal before your yoga practice: try to eat a small meal no less than two hours beforehand or, if you have eaten a large meal, then wait at least four hours before practising. If you need to eat more regularly you should seek medical advice.

• As in any sporting activity, it is important to warm the body up before practising yoga to protect you from strains and injury. Limbering up exercises are included on pages 17 to 31.

• The British Wheel of Yoga, which is recognised by the Sports Council as the governing body for yoga in Great Britain, does not recommend that pregnant women take up yoga and suggests waiting until a few weeks after the baby's birth. Neither is it recommended to practise yoga during the first trimester. However, there may be someone in your area who specialises in teaching yoga during pregnancy from whom you can seek advice.

• People with uncontrolled high blood pressure, heart disease or those suffering from serious eye problems such as glaucoma, should not practise inverted postures where the head is lower than the heart or vigorous postures such as those featured in the Warrior series, as they increase pressure in the thoracic cavity and the in eyes.

• During standing postures, those with heart problems and people with high or low blood pressure will need to be especially aware of how they are feeling, and gently come out of the posture and rest if necessary.

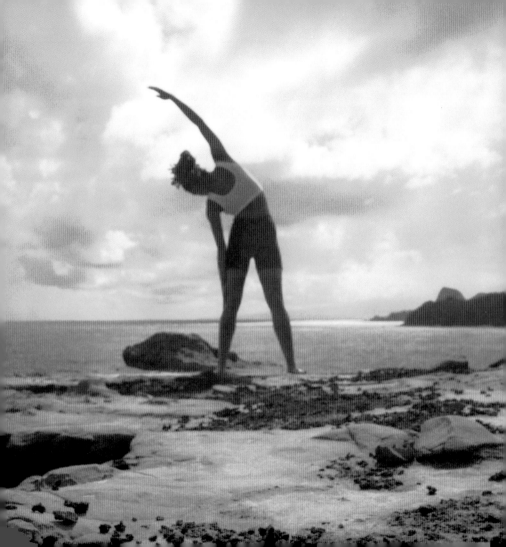

• Arthritis restricts mobility in the joints and often weakens them, and some asanas will not be comfortable for them. For example, practising the Cat pose (page 28) if you have weak wrists will be painful and may cause further damage, so should be avoided, as should kneeling postures for those who have arthritis in their knees.

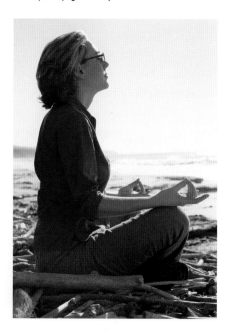

• People with varicose veins should be aware that the blood circulation can be cut off while kneeling.

• If you have a slipped disc then extreme caution should be used in forward bending. Backward and forward bends can also be uncomfortable for people with a gastric ulcer or hiatus hernia.

• It is important for everyone to avoid compressing the spine, especially when bending the head or back backwards. Working slowly with awareness, and using exhalation to feel the spine lengthen will help in avoiding compression of the vertebrae.

• Remember, if you feel uncomfortable or unwell in a posture, then carefully come out of it and rest.

What will I Need to Start off?

Taking up yoga doesn't have to cost a lot: you're likely to have everything you need to start at home already.

You need to have comfortable, non-restrictive, but not too baggy, clothing to allow the body to move freely. Remember that you may be raising the legs into the air – so jogging bottoms or leggings would be ideal, especially in a class situation.

You will need something to lie on – start off with a rug or blanket to see if you like yoga before spending money on a special yoga mat. A blanket may also come in useful if you feel cold during relaxation.

It is important to practice standing postures on a non-slip surface and if you are practising at home then probably your flooring will be fine, so long as you take off your socks.

A yoga belt is very useful in some postures to avoid having to over-stretch, a dressing gown belt could also be used.

You may find sitting on the floor uncomfortable, so, if you do not have a yoga block, use a plump cushion or a thick telephone directory to sit on.

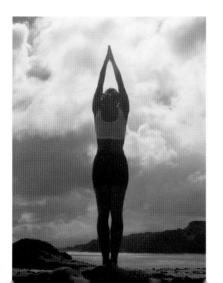

15

Practising at Home

A yoga session will include taking the body in all directions, i.e. forward, backward and lateral or sideways bending. There should be a spinal rotation or twist, a balance posture and an inverted posture. All the main joints should be exercised.

It is important to try to practise equally on each side. If, for example, you stretch through the right side of the body you should then stretch through the left side for the same length of time. This is referred to as a counter pose. By practising in this way you will bring balance to your body.

As you develop your yoga practice you may find that your body naturally seeks a counter pose after a strong asana. After a backward bend, for example, you may automatically hug the knees into the chest to take the spine in the other direction. Until this becomes automatic, make sure you consciously perform a counter pose. After an energetic asana it is good to come back to stillness by standing in Tadasana (page 42).

When coming out of a position, take your time and reverse the steps you used to go into the posture – this gives the body time to adjust and protects against injury, or dizziness when coming out of a head-down pose.

The asanas featured in this book have been grouped together into kneeling, sitting, standing, balancing, backward bending, forward bending, inverted and twisting postures. It is not the intention to perform all the asanas in one session, but rather, try to practise at least one posture from each section. Suggested sequences are on pages 100 to 103.

Warming-up

It's important to warm the body up before any exercise, so perform these lying down limbers to prepare the body for the work ahead.

1. Lie on your back in a straight line. As you inhale take the right arm overhead and at the same time stretch through to the right heel, flexing the foot (A). Slowly return the arm to your side on exhalation and relax the leg muscles. Repeat on the left side. Practise this exercise up to five times on each side, sometimes stretching through to the toes rather than the heel, but be aware that this can cause cramp. For a more gentle stretch keep the arms slightly bent.

2. Lying on your back with the legs bent, pick your feet up off the ground until the feet are in the air above your abdomen. Gently place the fingertips on each knee and draw the knees in circles taking them out to each side and then bringing them into the centre again. With the fingertips still guiding the knees take them apart and bring then back together again in circles. Repeat each knee circling method up to seven times in each direction.

3. Lie on your back with the legs bent and the feet flat on the floor and parallel. Have the hands resting on the abdomen and feel this area rise on inhalation and drop down on exhalation. Feel that the spine lengthens as you breathe out.

A.

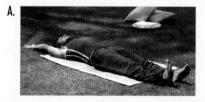

Let the arms rest alongside the body and encourage the back of the waist to make contact with the floor and then return to normal. Do this a couple of times, then allow the pelvis to lift very slightly off the floor (B). Very slowly let it come back into contact with the floor. Take your time and do not lift the pelvis too far off the floor as this exercise is intended as a gentle, stretching of the lower back and buttock muscles. Repeat five to seven times.

4. Another good warm up is to practice some cycling movements while lying on your back — remembering to do as many back pedals as forward ones!

5. For the hamstring stretch you need a belt or a tie. Lie on your back with the legs bent and the feet flat on the floor. Pick the right foot off the floor and hook the belt around the ball of the foot. Gently try to straighten the leg, being careful not to strain the leg or create tension in the shoulders (C). Try to work with the breath and feel that the body is opening with every out breath. In time you may find that the leg will straighten up quite easily but for others the knee will never be completely straight; the important thing is to never over-stretch or strain to get into a particular position. To lower the leg, bend it and then lower the foot to the floor. Repeat on the left side and try to hold the position as long as you did on the right side.

6. Lie on your back with the legs bent and feet a little apart for this gentle twisting exercise. Have the arms out at shoulder height. On the out breath let the knees drop down slowly to the right towards

B.

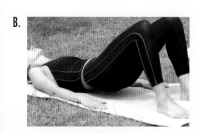

C.

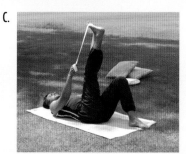

the floor, letting them float up to centre as you inhale. On the next exhalation let the knees drop to the left, again letting them float up to centre on the in breath. Try to keep the shoulder blades in contact with the floor. Complete up to seven times on each side. If you want to you can hold the posture for a few breaths or a count of twenty.

Note

It is always advisable to raise and lower your legs while they are bent as you can injure your back lifting and lowering straight legs.
This is due to their weight, and the effort required by the abdominal muscles, which may not be strong enough, thus making the back muscles take the strain.

Savasana or Corpse Pose

Savasana is the main pose for relaxation but it is also a great pose to include in your warming-up exercises.

1. Lie on the floor in a straight line, try to ensure that the spine is straight and the hips level. Have the legs a little apart and allow the feet to flop outwards. Rest the arms on the floor a little distance from the sides of the body, preferably with the palms facing the ceiling and the fingers curling naturally. The back of the neck should be long – tuck the chin in a little towards the chest and feel the back of the neck lengthen (A).

2. It is important to be comfortable in Savasana and if you feel that the back of your neck is shortening then have a folded towel or a yoga block under the head to raise it slightly. People with lower back problems may feel more comfortable with a pillow or rolled up towel under the backs of the knees.

The alternative posture for relaxation for those with lower back problems is to lie with the legs bent as described in semi-supine.

Semi-supine

Lie on your back and bend the legs, placing the feet flat on the floor. The feet should be about hip width apart and parallel, with the toes pointing forwards.

For relaxation, if it feels more comfortable, then you can let the knees rest against each other. The arms should be resting a little distance away from the sides of the body with the palms of the hands uppermost (B).

SUPINE LIMBERS

20

A.

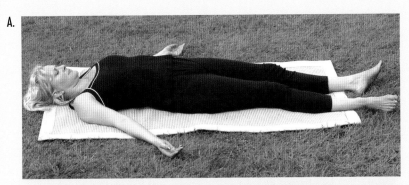

B.

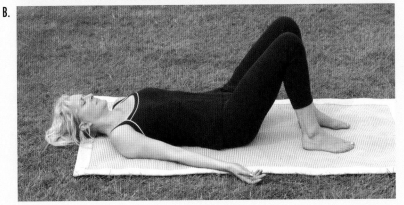

Limbering-up Exercises: Neck

*After completing the supine limbers
you can continue your warm-up
with these seated exercises, which
target more specific areas.
It is not necessary to perform all of
them nor in the order shown.*

Cautions:

People with neck or upper back problems should
always take great care when performing neck
exercises. Everyone must be especially careful
when taking the head back as it is very easy to
compress the vertebrae in the neck.
Taking the head back can cause problems and
you should not do it if you know you have a
neck condition or you experience any pain.

1. Sit or kneel in a comfortable position with the
spine straight. The shoulders should be relaxed and
dropping away from the ears, the chin parallel with
the floor (A). On the out breath turn the head
towards the right as far as is comfortable, bring the
head back to centre as you inhale, then as you
exhale, turn the head to the left, coming back to
centre as you breathe in. Repeat this exercise three
to five times, making sure that it is only the head
that moves (B).

2. Sitting as before, tilt the head to the right as you
exhale, so that the right ear moves towards the
right shoulder (C). Make sure that you do not lift
the shoulder to meet the ear! Return to the starting
position as you breath in. Tilt the head to the left on
exhalation, coming back to centre on inhalation.
Repeat this exercise three to five times. It will
stretch out the muscles down the sides of the neck.

A.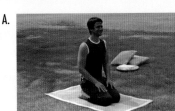

B.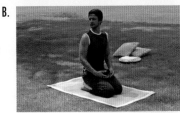

C.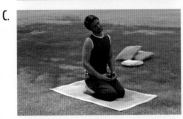

D.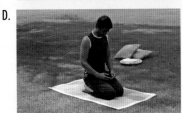

3. From the sitting position, allow the chin to slowly travel towards the chest as you breathe out, ensuring that you do not hunch your shoulders forwards with the chin (D). Return to the starting position as you breathe in and then repeat twice more.

4. Take the head back gently by following the eyes as they travel along the floor and up the wall in front of you, resting a moment when they reach the top of the wall (or sooner if you feel you need to). Then slowly follow the eyes as they travel a little along the ceiling directly in front of you. Be aware all the time of what is happening at the back of the neck and try to feel that it is lengthening with every exhalation.

Limbering-up Exercises: Shoulders

All shoulder limbers begin in a seated position although limbers 3 and 4 can also be done while lying down.

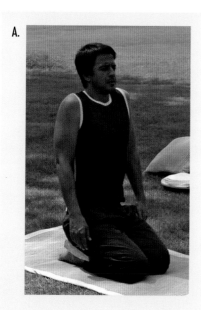

A.

1. Sitting in a comfortable position, slowly hunch the shoulders up towards the ears as you inhale and then gradually let them drop back down while you breathe out. Repeat the exercise (up to five times) seeing if you can exhale a little more and drop the shoulders further down each time (A).

2. Place the fingertips on the shoulders and slowly draw circles in the air with the elbows (B). Repeat up to seven times in each direction.

3. With the arms slightly bent, allow them to float upwards in a circular motion until they are above the head. Let them float down again in the same manner on exhalation. Repeat up to five times.

4. Rest the hands on your lap; on the in breath lift the arms in front of you until they are above the head. Let them float back down in front of you as you breathe out. Repeat up to five times.

B.

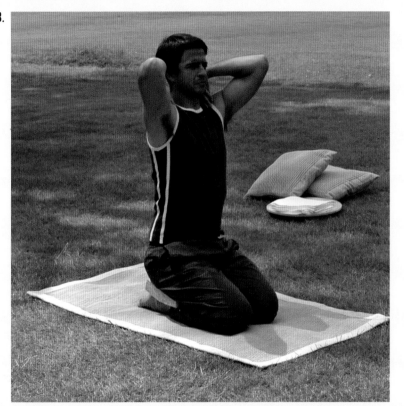

Limbering-up Exercises: Legs and Feet

All these exercises can be carried out while sitting in a straight-backed chair if sitting on the floor is uncomfortable.

1. Sit on the floor with the legs straight out in front of you in Dandhasana or the Staff Pose which is illustrated on page 37. Slowly tip the feet towards the floor, stretching the tops of the feet and the front of the lower leg, then draw them back up towards the shins, stretching the soles of the feet and the back of the lower leg. Try to keep the knees still. Repeat three to five times (A).

2. Taking the feet apart a little, slowly rotate the feet to exercise the ankles. Rotate up to seven times in each direction (B).

3. Bending the right leg, take hold of the lower part with the left hand and hold the back of the thigh with the right hand, then very gently circle the lower leg up to five times in each direction to warm up the knee joint (C). Repeat with the left leg.

A.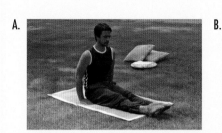

B.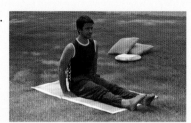

C.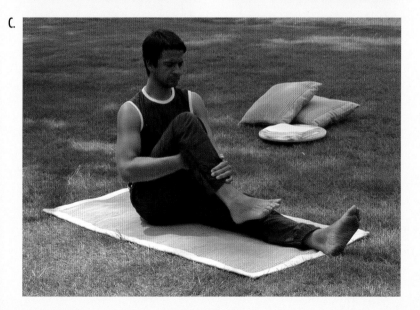

Majariasana or Cat Pose

*Majariasana and Apanasana
(page 30) are both yogic postures
but they are also used to warm
up the spinal area*

Caution:
Extra care should be taken if you have knee and wrist problems. With lower back problems do not dip the spine too low.

Benefits:
Improves flexibility of the spine, strengthens the arms and shoulders. May bring relief for menstrual cramps.

Modification:
Once you are familiar with the Cat, try changing the breathing so that you only move the spine as you exhale and breathe in while in the arched or concave position.

1. From a kneeling position go down on all fours, ensuring that the wrists are directly under the shoulders and the knees directly under the hips. The fingers should point forwards and the tops of the feet should be flat on the floor. The elbows should be straight throughout the practice (A).

2. Breathe in and at the same time drop the spine and abdomen down, taking the chest forward and raising the head (making sure you do not to take the head too far back and compress the neck) (B).

3. On an exhalation, lower the head and curl it into the chest while arching the spine like a cat (C).

Repeat the practice in a flowing manner, co-ordinating long, slow breaths with the movement.

A.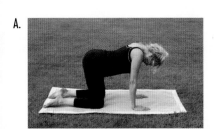

B.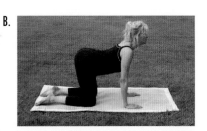

C.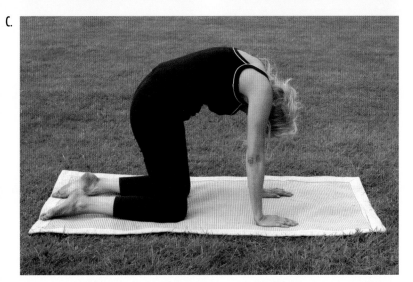

29

Apanasana

Caution:
Take great care and go gently if you have had a recent abdominal operation.

Benefits:
Strengthens the lower back muscles and massages the abdominal organs – this posture is sometimes referred to as the 'wind relieving posture'!

Modifications:
A more advanced way of practising Apanasana is by bringing both knees in towards the chest, remembering to lift the feet up one at a time. Provided there are no neck or upper back problems the head can be raised on the out breath and the chin taken towards the navel. Always lower the head back to the floor as you inhale (B).

1. Lie on the floor in the semi-supine position (page 20), and on an out breath, draw the right knee up towards the chest. If you have knee problems then it is better to take hold of the leg at the back of the thigh (A) otherwise you can link the fingers around the shin below the knee joint.

2. Release the leg slightly to breathe in, and then draw the knee back towards the chest on the next exhalation. Repeat twice more, before returning the right foot to the floor and repeating the asana on the left side.

3. Once you become familiar with this asana, and provided you have no lower back problems, you can practise it with the passive leg straight out on the floor.

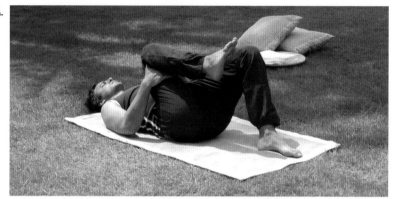

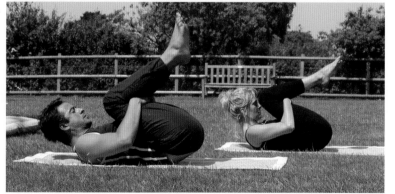

31

Vajrasana or Thunderbolt Pose

Caution:

People with varicose veins must be very careful as the circulation can be cut off. If you have knee problems then take great care when practising this posture.

Benefits:

This is a calming pose if practised with the eyes closed. It strengthens the legs, knees and pelvic area and is also said to benefit the digestive system.

Modification:

You may find it more comfortable to have a block or a folded blanket either between the buttocks and the feet or between the thighs and calves (A). Discomfort at the front of the foot may be alleviated by placing a folded towel underneath the foot.

1. Kneel on the floor, keeping the inside edges of the knees together and the big toes touching.

2. Allow the heels to open out and then lower the buttocks onto the 'seat' which is created by the undersides of the feet. The spine should be straight and the hands resting on the thighs. Close the eyes and breathe freely.

3. Try holding the posture for one minute before gradually building up the time spent in the posture. The neck and shoulder limbers shown on pages 22 to 25 can be practised while in Vajrasana.

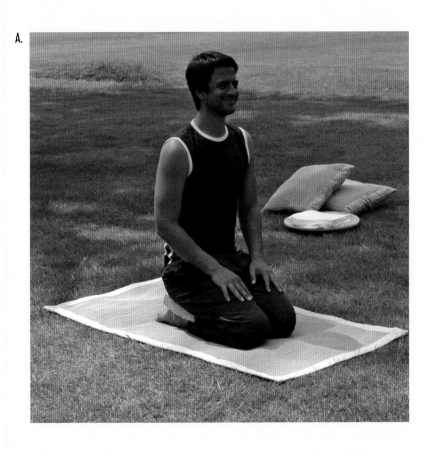

A.

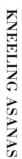

KNEELING ASANAS

Virasana or Hero's Pose

Caution:

This is a much stronger pose than Vajrasana and everyone should be careful to avoid straining the legs, particularly the knees. It should not be attempted if you have cartilage or ligament problems in the knees.

Modification:

If you are unable to keep the knees together, start off having the thighs parallel with the feet slightly wider apart. Then lower the buttocks between the feet.

1. Kneel on the floor with the knees touching but with the feet apart (A).

2. Slowly lower the buttocks onto the floor between the legs and feet. If the buttocks do not comfortably reach the floor, place a block lengthways between the legs (B).

A.
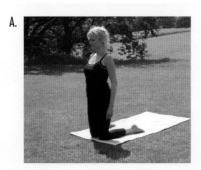

B.
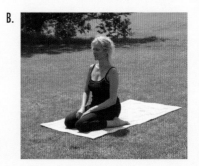

Supta Virasana or Reclining Hero Pose

Benefits:
This asana can be practised after eating as it is said to aid digestion.

1. Kneel as in Virasana (page 40).

2. Then, using the hands for support, carefully lower yourself backwards so that eventually you lie back between the legs (A).

To start off with you will probably need bolsters or folded blankets under the back for support. If you do use support under the spine make sure that the head is well supported, too.

A.

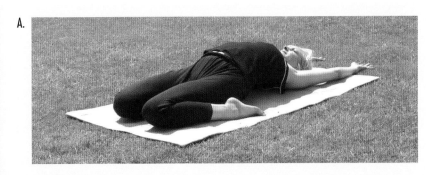

Swan and Child Poses

These are lovely poses for resting in after a strong asana, as they allow the spine to release and the breath to return to normal.

Caution:
People with heart problems, high blood pressure or eye conditions should not have the head lower than the heart, so either use a block or the fists one on top of the other under the forehead to keep the head raised. As with the other kneeling postures, be especially careful if you have varicose veins or knee problems.

Swan Pose
From a kneeling position, slowly bend forwards (using the hands for support) until the forehead rests on the ground. The arms should be outstretched in front of you with the palms resting on the floor (A). Feel the body widen as you breathe in and lengthen as you breathe out.

Child Pose
This is very similar to the Swan pose but the arms rest alongside the body with the hands by the feet (B).

A.
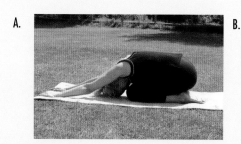

B.
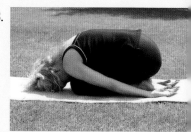

Dandasana or Staff Pose

*This pose is more difficult to
achieve than it looks!*

Benefits:
Dandasana helps to open the chest and
strengthens the arms, shoulders and back.

A.
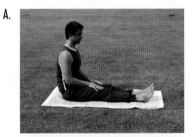

B.
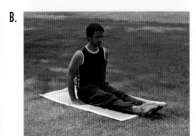

1. Sit on the floor with the legs touching and straight out in front of you (A).

2. Stretch through to the heels and keep the feet at right angles with the legs. The spine is straight, the back of the neck long, and the hands flat on the floor beside the hips, with the fingers pointing forwards.

3. Press gently down with the hands, keeping the shoulders back and dropping away from the ears. Feel the chest open (B).

4. Only maintain the pressure through the hands for a few seconds to begin with. Remember to breathe freely throughout the practice. You may sit on a block or a folded blanket for this posture.

Baddha Konasana or Cobbler's Pose

Caution:
Be very careful if you have sciatica or sacro iliac/sacrum problems as the posture does work on that area. Anyone with knee and hip problems should also take care.

Benefits:
Strengthens and tones the leg muscles, and exercises the hip joints. A good posture for menstrual and bladder problems.

1. Sit in Dandasana then bend the legs, taking the knees out to the sides so that the soles of the feet come together. Try to have the heels as close in to the pubis as possible, without straining the knees or hips by forcing the heels in too close. For added support this pose can be practised sitting against a wall.

2. If you can comfortably reach, link the fingers around the toes (A). Alternatively, hold on to the ankles or lower leg.

3. Carefully allow the knees to open out and drop towards the floor (B). Never force the knees down. Breathe freely and hold the pose for a minute or two, if comfortable. The more you practice, the longer you can remain in the posture.

A.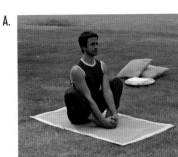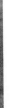

B.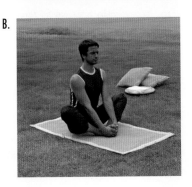

Don't be surprised if one knee lowers more than the other – to start with, you can support the knee(s) which does (do) not reach the ground on folded blankets.

4. A variation of Baddha Konasana is the Butterfly pose. In the Butterfly the knees move up and down in synchrony with the breath, resembling the wings of a butterfly. As you exhale, slowly lower the knees as far as they comfortably go and then let them slowly float up while you breathe in. Repeat a few times. The Butterfly can be practised as a warm up for Baddha Konasana.

Gomukhasana or Cowface Posture

This is quite a complex posture with challenging arm and leg positions. To start off with it is recommended that you concentrate on the arm position and only try the leg position after a few weeks.

Benefits:
Relieves backache and general stiffness in the shoulders and neck, and helps to open the chest. In the full pose, tension in the buttocks and lower back is relieved and the legs are toned. It is a great asana for inducing calmness.

The Arm Position

1. Sit or stand in a comfortable position. Stretch the right hand up, trying to feel the ribs opening up on the right side of the chest, (A) then bend the elbow and drop the hand behind the shoulder. The palm should be touching the back.

2. Draw a big circle with the left hand just below shoulder height, bending the elbow and taking the hand behind the back, with the palm facing out (B).

3. Slide this hand up the spine until you can clasp the fingers of both hands together (C). Hold the posture for thirty seconds to begin with and

A.

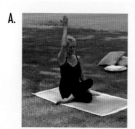

B.

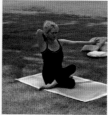

C.

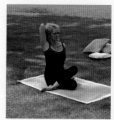

remember to breathe freely throughout. Repeat with the left arm up and over and the right arm around the back (D). In the full position the fingers link behind the back, but if you can't do this, have a belt in the hand that goes up and over so you can take hold of it with the other hand (E).

In this posture the spine should remain upright with the raised upper arm behind the ear. However, the tendency can be to bend forwards to bring the ear in front of the arm and you should try to avoid doing this. Be careful not to twist the arms to clasp the hands together.

The Leg Position

1. Sit with the legs out in front of you and then cross the left leg over the right, bending the leg so that the left foot rests alongside the right hip.

2. Bend the right leg and bring the foot around to the left so that it rests beside your left hip. In this pose one knee is directly on top of the other (see page 40). With the left leg on top you should have the right arm as the upper arm, and vice versa. Remember to change the leg position when you change the arm position. If your hips are stiff then the bottom leg can remain straight.

D.

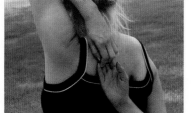

E.

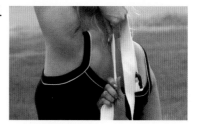

41

Tadasana or Mountain Pose

Tadasana is the basic standing pose and all other standing poses start with it. The great thing about Tadasana is that you can practise it anywhere.

1. Stand with the feet slightly apart, ensuring that the feet are parallel. A good way of checking if the feet are parallel is to see if the second toes are pointing straight ahead.

2. Imagine three roots growing out of each foot — one from the base of the big toe, another from the base of the little toe and the third through the centre of the heel. Send the weight of your body evenly through each of these points in the feet. If you are unsure, without moving the feet, take the weight forwards slightly and then backwards before bringing the weight to centre again to find the point where it is evenly distributed through the feet.

3. The legs should be straight but not locked at the knees. The shoulders should be relaxed and dropping away from the ears, with the arms hanging softly at each side. The chest should feel open throughout the practice (A).

4. Be aware of your breathing and try to feel that the spine lengthens with every exhalation. With this lengthening the coccyx at the very end of the spine drops down and tucks under.

5. The back of the neck is long and the crown of the head is parallel with the ceiling. There is no effort to hold the head in position.

This posture brings quietness and balance back to the body and mind and should be practised for thirty to sixty seconds to begin with. Remember though, if you have heart or blood pressure problems you may need to come out of the posture sooner than this.

A.

Simple Shoulder Release Pose

Caution:

Do not practise this if you have an acute problem with your shoulder joints.

Benefits:

Opens the chest, strengthens the upper back and shoulders and releases tension in these areas.

1. Stand with the feet parallel and about 30 cm apart. Bring the hands to the Namaste (prayer) position (A) at the heart centre (page 115) – have the forearms parallel with the floor and the elbows pointing out to the sides.

2. As you breathe in, take the hands out to the sides in big circles and around to the back (B).

3. On the out breath link the fingers behind the back and let the hands drop down as you straighten the arms. You should feel the shoulders moving back and the chest open as you take a couple of breaths in this position.

4. On an inhalation, and with the hands still linked behind you, lift the arms up as high as comfortable. Take care not to lean forwards when doing this.

5. As you breathe out let the hands slowly return to the back of the pelvis (C), and take a couple of recovery breaths before repeating once or twice more.

At the end of the practice release the hands and stand in Tadasana for a moment or two.

A.

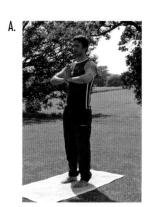

B.

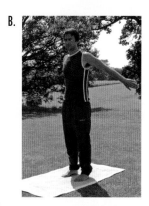

C.

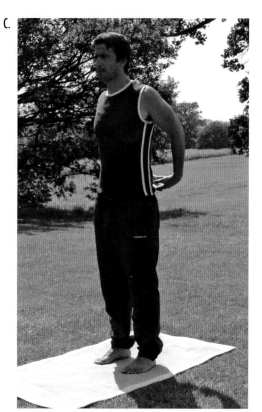

45

Parsvottanasana or Flank Stretch

Caution:
Be sure not to strain to get into this pose. Those with blood pressure, heart or eye problems should take care in this standing, forward-bend pose.

Benefits:
Relieves stiffness in the hips and leg muscles, helps to improve flexibility in the wrists and shoulders, corrects rounded shoulders and tones the abdominal organs.

Reverse Namaste

1. In Parsvottanasana the hands are held in Namaste at the back of the body (A).

2. To do this, bring the hands around to the back, palms together, fingers pointing down. Then turn the hands upwards and slide them up between the shoulder blades, taking the shoulders back.

3. If you are not able to do this then try having the back of one hand touching the area between the shoulder blades with the back of the other hand on top of it (B). An alternative is to have the arms folded at the back of the waist (C).

A.
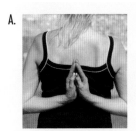

B.
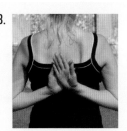

C.
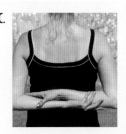

A.

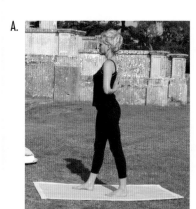

B.

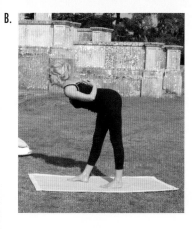

Parsvottanasana

1. Stand with the feet hip width apart and the hands in Namaste at the back.

2. Take a step forwards with the right foot, keeping the weight evenly through both feet (A).

3. Inhale, feeling the body open and expand, then as you exhale, bend forwards from the hips keeping the weight through the back foot as the stretch through the front leg intensifies. Try not to tilt the head or hunch the shoulders to bring them closer to the front leg (B). The back of the pelvis should be level. Hold the posture for up to thirty seconds, breathing freely through the nose before slowly coming up on an inhalation.

4. Take a step back to align the feet again. Then repeat with the left foot forward. Afterwards, ease out the shoulders with gentle rotations.

47

Trikonasana or Triangle Pose

Caution:
Take care not to over-stretch the lower back if you tend to suffer from problems in this area.

Benefits:
Regular practice of Trikonasana will tone the entire body, particularly the sides and the legs, and help reduce fat around the waistline. The abdominal organs are massaged and this helps to improve digestion.

Modification:
If the knees feel over-stretched, slightly bend the knee on the side you are taking the body to.

1. From Tadasana take a step to the side so that the feet are about a leg's length apart. Turn the right foot 90° out to the right and bring the left toes in slightly. The hips should remain facing forwards (A).

2. As you breathe in, float the arms up from the sides until they are at shoulder height (B). As you exhale feel the arms lengthen and the shoulders release. Sense the triangles that your body is forming and try to feel the energy in them.

3. On an out breath bend the body to the right until the right hand comes lightly into contact with the right leg. The left arm should rise, so that the arms form a straight line. The left palm should be facing forwards. If there are no neck problems you can turn the head to look up at the top hand. Hold the posture for up to thirty seconds, breathing freely (C).

A.

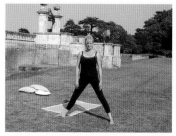

B.

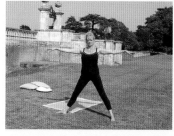

C.

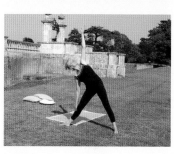

4. To come out of the posture, turn the head to the centre, breathe in as you raise the body upright and exhale as you slowly lower the arms to the sides of the body and bring the feet to face forwards again. Repeat on the left side.

Note

More flexible people can reach their foot or the floor with the right hand without twisting the body to get the hand down that far. Be aware of keeping the left hip back and facing forwards as you bend to the right to ensure that you don't twist. A good test for this is to stand with the back against a wall and as you bend to the right, keep the back in contact with the wall — you will probably find that you don't get so far down the leg, but in this way you are working the intended muscles properly.

Virabhadrasana or Warrior Poses

The three postures in the Warrior series are strenuous, but energising.

Caution:
It is not recommended that people with uncontrolled high blood pressure, any type of heart problem or serious eye conditions should attempt these asanas.

Benefits:
Helps to improve breathing as the chest is open, relieves stiffness in the shoulders and back, and strengthens the legs and ankles.

Virabhadrasana 1

1. Stand in Tadasana and then take the feet wide apart (wider than for Trikonasana) (A).

2. Turn the right foot out to the right by 90° and turn the left toes in slightly – the right heel should be in line with the arch of the left foot. Turn the body to face over the right leg. On inhalation, bring the arms up overhead with the upper arms alongside the ears. The hands can remain parallel or you can bring the palms together (B).

3. On an exhalation, bend the right knee, keeping the left leg straight and the outer edge of the left

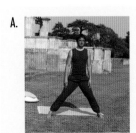 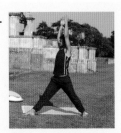 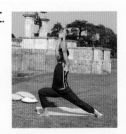

A. B. C.

foot in contact with the floor. In the full pose the right knee will be directly over the right heel, with the shin perpendicular to the floor and the right thigh parallel with the floor (C).

The knee should never extend over the right toes as this takes the knee out of alignment. If this happens, you will need to bring the knee back until it is in line with the heel even if it means that the thigh is no longer parallel with the floor (see note below). Breathe freely and relax into the posture for a few seconds, feeling that the spine is lengthening.

4. To come out of the pose, inhale as you straighten the right knee and exhale as you lower the arms to the sides. Repeat on the left side.

Note
Next time you practice the pose, take the feet wider apart so long as you do not feel that you are going to overbalance.

Virabhadrasana 2
Benefits:
Strengthens and tones the leg and back muscles and tones the abdominal organs.

1. As with the first Warrior pose, take the feet wide apart and turn the right foot out to the right side by 90° and turn the left toes inwards slightly (right heel in line with left instep).

2. Inhale and let the arms float up to shoulder height with the palms of the hands pointing down. Keep the body facing forwards (A).

A.

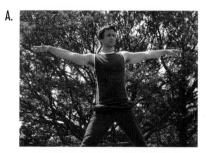

Virabhadrasana or Warrior Poses continued

3. On an exhalation bend the right knee as in Virabhadrasana 1. The arms should remain at shoulder height and outstretched to the sides. Turn to look down the right arm (B). Hold the posture for up to thirty seconds breathing freely.

4. To come out of the pose, inhale as you straighten the right knee and exhale as you lower the arms to the sides. Repeat on the left side.

B.
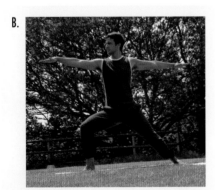

Virabhadrasana 3

This is the most difficult of the Warrior series as it is a balance starting from Virabhadrasana 1.

Caution:
Take care that the standing leg is not over-extended by having the straight knee pushed back and locked.

1. Starting with the right side first, come into Virabhadrasana 1. Hold the posture for a breath or two.

2. Then as you exhale, bend the torso forwards over the bent leg, keeping the arms straight out in front of you. The palms can be touching or a little distance apart (A). Hold this position for a couple of breaths.

3. On an exhalation, push away from the floor with the left foot, leaning further forwards and at the same time straightening the right leg (B). It can be helpful in this balance to have the hands a little apart, imagining that you are clasping a tree trunk.

4. In the full posture the left leg is parallel with the floor; in fact your whole body (apart from the supporting leg) should be parallel with the floor. Hold the posture for up to thirty seconds, breathing freely.

5. The traditional way to come out of the posture is to return to Virabhadrasana 1 and then straighten the leg and lower the arms as described earlier. An alternative method is to lower the hands to the floor, resting on the fingertips, bend the supporting knee and bring the raised leg down beside the other. Spend a moment or two in this position before slowly coming up to standing. Repeat on the other side.

Counter pose

A counter pose for these asanas is to come into Utthanasana, or the standing forward bend which is described on page 56.

A.

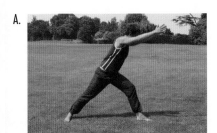

B.

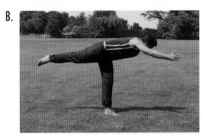

Parsvakonsasana or Side Angle Pose

Benefits:
Tones the ankles and legs. Reduces fat around the waist and hips and may help relieve sciatic and arthritic pains. Helps the digestive process.

1. Stage one – from Tadasana take the feet quite wide apart and turn the right foot out 90° and the left toes in slightly. On an in breath, float the arms up to shoulder height. Continue to face forwards (A).

2. Bend the left leg on an exhalation and lower the torso down onto the bent leg, resting the left forearm across the left thigh (B). The right arm is now pointing up towards the sky. Provided you do not have neck or shoulder problems look up at the outstretched arm (C).

3. As you breathe, feel that the spine is lengthening and the body opening and allow the right arm to travel over the head, so that the whole of the right side of the body from foot to fingertips is in a lovely straight line. Ensure that the left knee does not extend beyond the toes. Hold the posture for up to thirty seconds to begin with.

4. Repeat on the other side with the right leg bent and the stretch through the right side of the body. Once you have mastered stage one you can move onto stage two.

5. Stage two – bend the left leg on an exhalation, lowering the torso onto the bent leg. This time place the left hand flat on the floor on the inside of the left foot (D). If you cannot reach the floor, use a block or two to rest the hand on.

6. As with stage one, the right arm points straight up (E) and then moves across with the exhalations. Turn the head to look up. In this stage the stretch through the side of the body is more intense. Repeat on the other side.

A.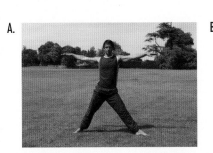

B.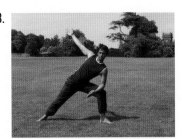

C.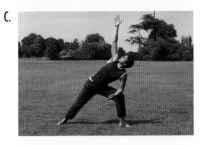

D.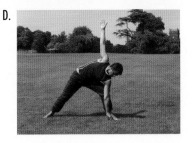

E.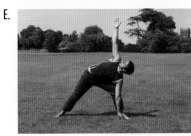

Utthanasana or Standing Forward Bend

Caution:

Do not attempt this posture if you have sciatica or other back problems – practice the alternative (Rag Doll) version described on the following page instead. Utthanasana may be uncomfortable for those with hiatus hernia. As this is a head down posture, people with uncontrolled high blood pressure, heart or serious eye problems should practice it by placing the hands on a window ledge or chair back so that the heart and the head remain level.

Benefits:

Massages the abdominal organs, increases blood flow to the brain. Stretches and strengthens the spine, stretches the hamstrings. Energises the whole body.

Modification:

Have the hands on the hips when bending forwards and also when coming back up.

1. Stand in Tadasana. On an inhalation, take the arms overhead so that the upper arms are alongside the ears (A).

2. On the exhalation, bend forwards from the hips, keeping the spine straight (B). Bend as far as you comfortably can without straining, resting the hands against the front of each leg if they don't reach the floor (C).

3. In the full (advanced) pose the chest touches the thighs and the head rests against the shins, with the hands flat on the floor. Remain in the posture for up to thirty seconds, breathing freely.

4. To come up, bring the arms alongside the ears, and slowly lift back up to the upright position. On an exhalation, let the arms float down to the sides of the body.

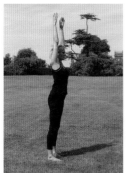

C.
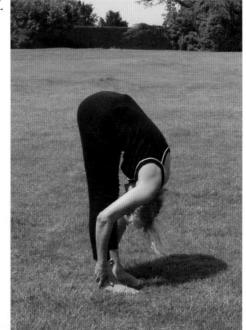

B.
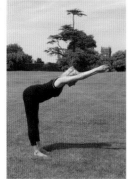

STANDING ASANAS

Alternative Standing Forward Bend or Rag Doll

This is a great 'undoing' pose and can be practised after a strenuous pose such as Virabhadrasana or Trikonasana.

Modification:

If you have a bad back or can't bend, only bend half-way down and place the hands on a chair back or window ledge (D). Try taking the feet slightly wider apart than in Tadasana. If you have sciatica, position the heels slightly out and the toes in.

1. Stand in Tadasana and bend the knees.

2. Slowly bend forwards, starting from the head and taking the chin towards the chest. Then bend the upper body, letting the shoulders roll forwards and the arms go limp (A).

3. Continue slowly bending the body forwards – like a rag doll with no spine (B). Let the arms hang loosely, folding them if they reach the ground.

4. Keeping the knees bent, let the body hang loosely but do not swing the torso around or force the body down further (C).

5. To come up, dip the buttocks down by bending the knees a little bit more, then slowly uncurl the spine, finishing with straightening the neck to bring the head up.

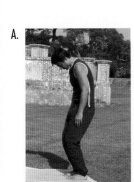
A.

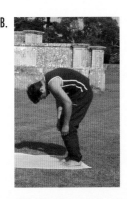
B.

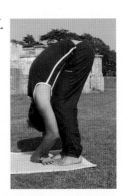
C.

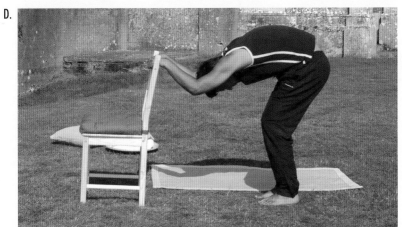
D.

Balancing Postures

As we get older, our ability to balance lessens so it is important to practise balancing poses, which not only help us physically but also bring about an emotional and spiritual equilibrium. Balancing also strengthens the leg muscles and improves concentration.

Modification:

In Vrksasana, if the raised foot does not reach the top of the opposite thigh, rest it lower down the leg. Take care if you rest the foot on the inside of the opposite knee that you do not push that knee out of alignment. The heel of the raised foot can also be rested on the ankle bone of the balancing foot, with the toes just touching the floor. Practice against a wall if you find it hard to balance, or you may prefer to only practice this part first while holding on to a chair back.

Vrksasana or Tree

1. Stand in Tadasana for a few moments to still the body and mind.

2. Gradually send the weight through the right foot and when you feel rooted, lift up the left foot and place the heel at the top of the inside left thigh with the toes pointing down. (This may not be possible for beginners and you should perform one of the modifications until flexibility improves.) The left knee should be pointing to the side and not the front (A).

3. Bring the hands to Namaste at your heart centre, pushing the palms together slightly. Breathe freely. Focus the gaze softly on a point in front of you (B).

4. If you feel strong and steady you can move to the next stage. Raise the arms overhead; keep the palms together and the elbows out and back (C).

5. Hold the pose for thirty seconds or so and very gradually work up to holding for about two minutes. To come out of the posture, bring the hands down to the sides and then release the raised foot back to the floor. Stand in Tadasana for a breath or two before repeating on the left foot. Practice Utthanasana or Rag Doll (page 58), or the Child pose (page 36) after balancing.

A.

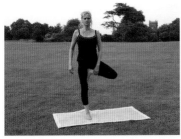

B.

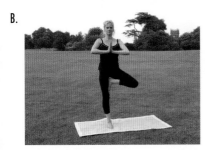

C.

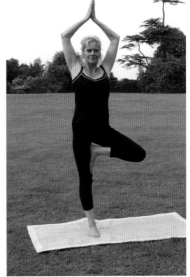

Natarajasana or Dancer Pose

Caution:
The full pose should not be attempted by those with recent, or chronic, injury to the legs, hips, back or shoulders.
Modification:
To give a feeling of security during balancing, stand with the side of the body with the outstretched arm close to the wall. Place the back foot on a chair and take the arm around the back of the waist.
In Stage 1, having caught hold of the back foot and raised the front hand, take the front hand around to take hold of the back foot, so that you are holding it in both hands. This intensifies the stretch through the quadriceps of the raised leg and takes the shoulders back, opening the chest.

1. Stage one – stand in Tadasana, then take the weight on to the right foot (A).

2. Bend the left leg and take the foot back while taking the left arm out and around to the back to take hold of the ankle. Try to keep the knees close together and the hips aligned (B).

3. The straight right arm floats forward and up so that the fingertips point diagonally to the ceiling (C). If you do not have a neck problem you can look up at the right hand, otherwise softly fix the gaze on a point on the floor in front of you. Practice this regularly on both sides before moving on the to the next stage.

4. Stage two – push the left foot away from you taking care not to swing the knee out of alignment (D). At this point allow the body to move forwards at the hips with the right arm coming forwards and down a little.

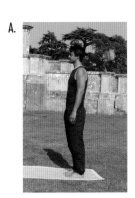

A.

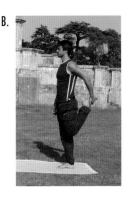

B.

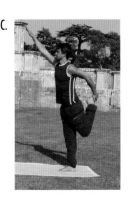

C.

5. A slight back bend has now been introduced. Again, master this before attempting to go into the full pose.

6. Stage three – the pose can be taken a step further by pushing the back foot even higher and drawing it closer to the back of the head. This is a very strong balance and back extension and should not be attempted by people with back, neck, shoulder, hip or leg problems.

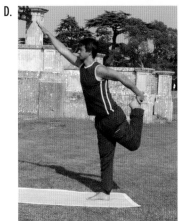

D.

Garudasana or Eagle Balance

Caution:
Do not strain to get into the full arm and leg positions.

Benefits:
Strengthens the muscles, tones the nerves, loosens the leg and arm joints. Relieves sciatica, rheumatism and hydrocele.

Modification:
If you find it very difficult to concentrate on the leg and arm positions, then practise each one separately until you feel confident enough to attempt the full posture.

1. Stand in Tadasana and then bend both legs. Lift up the left leg and cross it in front of the right thigh (A).

2. Wrap the left foot behind the right calf with the toes pointing down (B). To start off with you can have the left toes resting on the floor behind the right calf to give a sense of balance.

3. Now cross the arms in front of you with your left arm under the right (C). Twist the forearms around each other and try to bring the palms together. If you have short arms you will find this difficult! Breathe freely in the pose and hold for up to thirty seconds to begin with.

4. To come out of the posture, slowly undo the arms and legs and return to Tadasana. Repeat on the other side and remember to cross the right arm under the left when balancing on the left foot.

BALANCING ASANAS

64

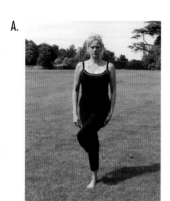

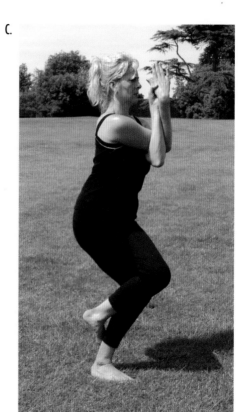

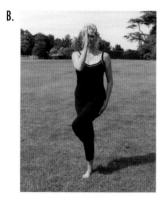

BALANCING ASANAS

65

Backbends: Sphinx

This is a good posture for stiff backs. Even those with acute backache or a slipped disc may practice it as long as they do not experience any discomfort.

1. Lie face down on the floor with the forehead resting on the floor. The legs are straight with the soles uppermost and the feet either touching or very slightly apart. The arms stretched out in front of you with the palms facing down (A).

2. Now slowly 'walk' the hands back towards the shoulders, bending the elbows. As you do this the forehead and chest will lift away from the floor.

3. Bring the elbows back until they are in line with the shoulder joints. Rest the forearms on the floor with your fingers pointing forwards (B).

4. Focus on the breath and try to feel the spine lengthening with every exhalation. The shoulders should be relaxed and dropping away from the ears. Feel that the thoracic area of the spine between the shoulder blades is becoming more supple with every breath. Hold the pose for up to two minutes.

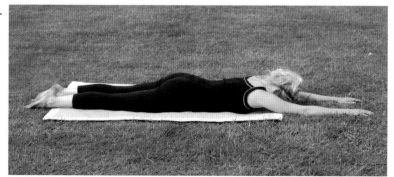

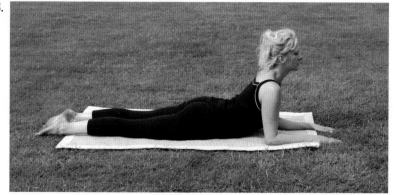

Bhujangasana or Cobra Pose

Caution:

Be very careful not to compress the spine in the lumbar area. Take care if you have weak or arthritic wrists or shoulders. People with a peptic ulcer or a hernia should seek medical advice before attempting this posture.

Benefits:

Strengthens the back muscles and can be helpful in cases of slipped disc. Increases flexibility of the spine, and strengthens the arms and pectoral muscles in the chest.

1. Lie face down on the floor and have the hands flat on the floor either side of the face, with the fingers pointing forwards (A). Focus on the breath and feel that the spine is opening and lengthening with every outward breath.

2. Slowly raise the head and chest away from the floor as you straighten the arms, but try to use the back muscles rather than just the arm muscles to lift up. Be aware the whole time of how the back is feeling. Ensure that you do not push up too high and compress the lower back. The degree of flexibility in the spine will dictate whether or not the elbows straighten. Keep the pubic bone in contact with the floor throughout this practice.

3. Relax the shoulders down from the ears and look straight ahead (B). Avoid taking the head back and risking injury to the neck. Hold the position for up to thirty seconds to begin with while breathing freely and focusing on lengthening the spine.

4. To come out of the posture, slowly bend the arms and lower the chest and head to the floor again. Rest with the face to one side before repeating once more if you wish.

A.

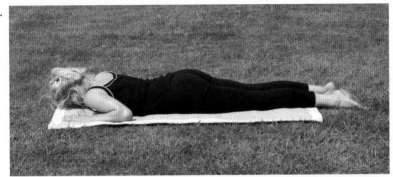

B.

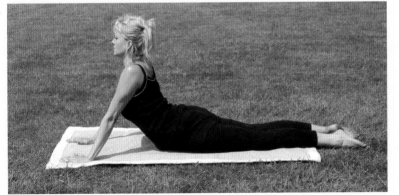

Salabhasana or Locust

This is a strong pose and it is recommended that the beginner works on Ardha Salabhasana (half locust) before attempting to practice the full posture.

Caution:

Those with heart problems or uncontrolled high blood pressure should not attempt the full asana. Nor is it suitable for those with a hernia or a peptic ulcer.

Modifications:

To assist with lifting the legs further from the floor, make fists with the hands and slip them under the groin, then lift the legs. An alternative is to place a block under the thighs. To provide more protection for the lower back, once the legs are lifted off the floor, stretch through to the heels. Release the stretch through the heels to lower the legs again.

Benefits:

Strengthens the lower back and aids backache and sciatica. The abdominal organs are toned.

1. In the classical pose the chin is resting on the floor while lying face down but it is recommended that you lie with the forehead on the floor as this keeps the back of the neck long and protects it from injury.

2. Position the arms alongside the body with the fingers pointing towards the feet with the legs together or very slightly apart (A). Spend a moment or two breathing freely and feeling the opening and lengthening of the spine.

3. Breathe in and lift the legs from the floor as high as you can while pushing gently into the floor with the hands (B). The toes are pointing straight back. Hold for up to thirty seconds, breathing freely. On an out breath slowly lower the legs to the floor.

A.

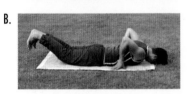

Ardha Salabhasana
or Half Locust

1. Lie face down as described for the full Locust pose, then breathing in, raise one leg only (C).

B.

2. Stretch through to the heel with the raised leg and hold the pose for up to thirty seconds breathing freely. Practice two or three times to each side.

C.

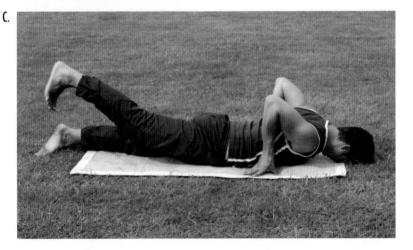

Matsyasana or Fish Pose

*This is an advanced posture
and should not be attempted until
the modified versions (opposite)
have been mastered.*

Caution:
Those with heart problems, ulcer, hernia, or back
or neck problems should not attempt the full
posture, and must also take care when
attempting the modified versions.

Benefits:
Opens the chest and encourages deep breathing,
benefits the thyroid gland, strengthens the hip
joints, stretches and tones the abdominal organs.

1. Sit in Padmasana (page 118) and then carefully take the body back using the arms and elbows for support (A).

2. Arching the back and opening the chest, bring the crown of the head to rest gently on the floor, ensuring that it is not pushing into the ground and putting strain on the neck (B).

3. To come out of the posture, use the arms for support and slide the head back and straighten the spine so that you are lying flat on the floor. As you breathe in come up to a sitting position and then release the legs.

Counter pose
After practising any version of Matsyasana, either rest for a while in Child pose (page 36) or sit with bent legs and gently lower the torso forwards to rest against the thighs to stretch out the back.

A.

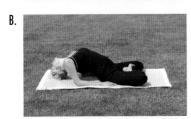

B.

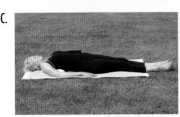

C.

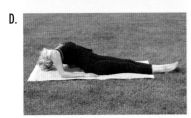

D.

Modified Fish 1

Roll up a towel or small blanket and place across your mat. Lie back so that it is directly under the shoulder blade area of the spine. The back of the head should be flat on the floor, and the legs in a straight line (C). Spend a couple of minutes in the pose, breathing freely. To come out of the pose, roll over to one side and remove the towel.

Modified Fish 2

Lie on your back, your hands flat on the floor (palms down and fingers facing the feet) just under each buttock. Inhale and arching the back, lift the head, shoulders and upper arms off the floor, taking the weight through the forearms and hands. On an exhalation, gently lower the crown of the head back onto the ground (D). Breathe freely and hold the pose for up to two minutes. Keep the weight through the arms then come out of the pose by sliding the head back until the back is flat on the floor. Gently push back up to sitting.

Setu Bandha Sarvangasana or Bridge Pose

Caution:
Take great care if you have knee problems. Not recommended for serious abdominal problems. Do not practice with a block or a cushion under the head.

Benefits:
Strengthens the legs, flexes the spine and opens the chest.

Modification:
Once in the full posture, link the fingers together behind the back and stretch the hands away towards the feet. This will help to dome the chest and lift the body a little higher.

Counter pose
As a counter pose, draw the knees into the chest taking hold of the backs of the thighs and very gently rock from side to side.

1. Lie on the back with the legs bent, arms alongside the body, feet flat on the floor, hip width apart and parallel, with the backs of the heels fairly close to the buttocks (A) (as in the pelvic tilt included within the limbering up section, page 18).

2. Ensure the weight is evenly distributed through the three points in each foot throughout the posture. In the final position the shins should be perpendicular to the floor.

3. Spend a little time focusing on the breath and feeling the spine lengthen. Check that the back of the neck is long.

4. Gradually lift the pelvis up off the floor (as you did in the pelvic tilt) and then slowly lower it down again. Repeat this a few times, taking the pelvis a little higher each time. All through the posture, be aware of the breath and the lengthening of the spine.

5. Slowly lift the pelvis and spine off the floor as high as is comfortable without straining, sending the weight through the three points in each foot (B). The knees move forwards. Remain in the pose for up to two minutes, breathing freely.

6. To come out of the posture, very slowly lower the spine, vertebra by vertebra back to the floor. Try to come down on the exhalation, stopping to breathe in and then lowering slowly again. Repeat once more after taking a few recovery breaths.

A.

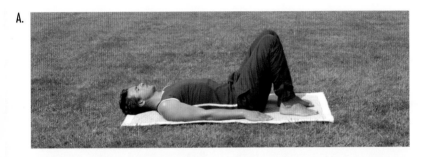

B.

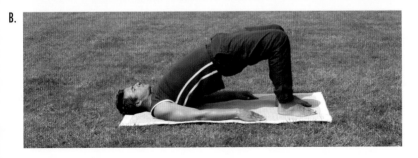

Forward Bending

Forward bends are relaxing and introverting and should be included towards the end of a yoga session to prepare for pranayama and relaxation.

Simple Version

This is an easy and calming forward bend which allows the spine to open up without any effort.

1. Sit with the legs bent and the feet flat on the floor, hip width apart.

2. Slowly bend the torso forwards to the thighs. Rest the hands on the shins or ankles and let the head hang loosely (A). Alternatively, if it feels more comfortable, cross the arms over the knees to rest the head on.

A.

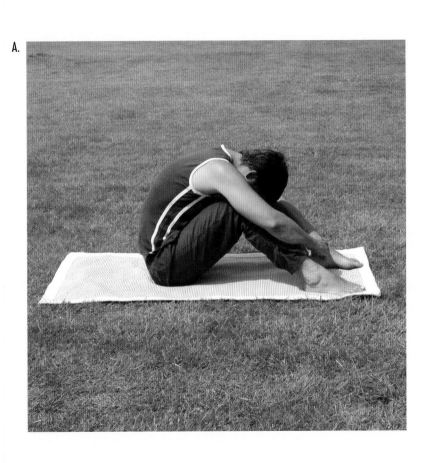

Paschimottanasana or Sitting Forward Bend

Caution:

Extreme care should be taken by people with a slipped disc or sciatica and it is recommended that they seek expert advice before attempting this asana.

Benefits:

Massages and tones the abdominal organs improving digestion, and also stretches the hamstrings and the back.

Modifications:

Have the legs slightly bent at the knees to lessen the stretch through the hamstrings.

Loop a belt or tie around the balls of the feet and lower down while holding on to the ends of it, but being careful that you are not creating tension in the shoulders by pulling on the belt (D).

Sit on a block or folded blanket, which will help when bending forwards. Rest the forehead on a block or folded blanket across the legs (E).

1. Sit on the floor in Dandasana but have the hands resting on the thighs (A).

2. Take a couple of breaths before bending the body forwards on an exhalation, keeping the spine as straight as possible and sliding the hands down the legs (B).

3. Try to take hold of the feet but if this is not possible then take hold of the ankles or any part of the leg which you can reach without straining (C). Remain in this position, breathing freely for a moment or two.

4. As you exhale, try to lower the torso closer to the legs, bending the elbows as you do so, but avoiding creating tension in the arms and shoulders. Breathe freely and hold this position for up to thirty seconds to begin with.

5. To come out of the pose, breathe in and slide the hands back up the legs as you bring the body back to the upright position.

A.

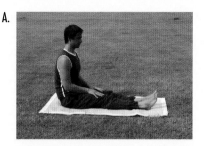

B.

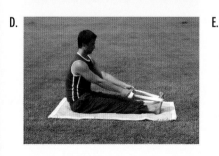

C.

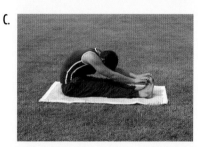

D.

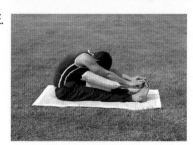

E.

Janu Sirsasana or Head to Knee Pose

Caution:

The same warnings apply as for Paschimottanasana (page 78). Great care should be taken by people with knee problems.

Benefits:

Similar to Paschimottanasana, with the added benefit of loosening up the legs.

Modification:

To keep the pelvis level, sit on a block or folded blanket (C); this will also help with bending forwards. If the bent knee doesn't reach the ground, support it on a folded blanket or block.

Use a belt around the ball of the foot as in Paschimottanasana. Rest the head on a block or folded blanket on the inside of the straight leg.

1. Sit on the floor with the legs straight out in front (A) and then bend the right leg, placing the sole of the right foot against the inside of the left thigh, with the heel as close to the perineum as possible. The outside of the knee should be resting on the floor. The left leg is straight and the foot is vertical with the toes pointing directly upwards (B). Breathe freely, trying to focus on the opening and lengthening of the spine.

2. On an out breath, bend forward from the hips, letting the hands glide down either side of the left leg. Keep the spine straight and head central, without straying over to the straight leg. Hold the pose for a moment or two, breathing freely (C).

3. To come up, breathe in and slowly come back up. Take a couple of deep breaths before practising the pose on the other side.

A.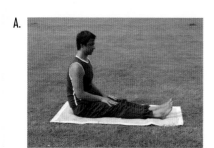

B.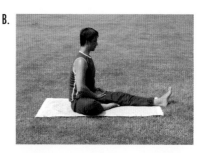

C.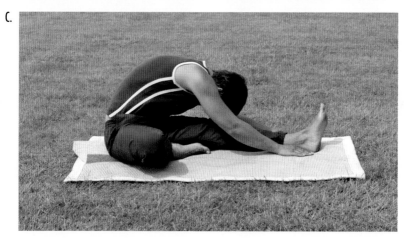

Upavista Konasana or Wide Angle Sitting Forward Bend

Caution:
As for Paschimottanasana (page 78).
Benefits:
As for Paschimottanasana (page 78).

Method 1

1. Sit up straight with your legs in front of you, then spread them wide apart, stretching through to the heels, feet vertical and toes pointing straight up (A). Sit on a block or folded blanket to assist in the bending forward if necessary.

2. Place the palms on the floor midway between the legs. As you breathe out, slide the hands forwards, bringing the torso down towards the floor between the legs (B). Take a couple of breaths before coming back up as you inhale. Repeat once more.

A.

B.

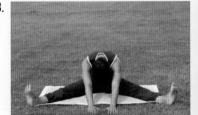

Method 2

1. Sit as in Method 1 with the legs wide apart, but turn the body over the right leg, placing the hands lightly on the right thigh or either side of the leg(C). On an out breath, slide the hands down the leg, bending from the hips (D). Take a breath or two before gently coming back up on an in breath.

2. Turn the body over the left leg and repeat. You can then take the body directly forwards as in Method 1.

C.
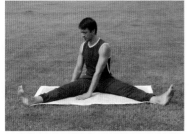

D.
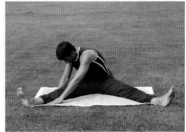

Adho Mukha Svanasana or Downward Facing Dog

Caution:
As this is a head down pose, people with uncontrolled high blood pressure, heart problems or serious eye problems should practice the modified version. Care should be taken by anyone with weak wrists.

Benefits:
Strengthens the arms and legs, tones and stimulates circulation in the upper back.

Modification:
If a head down pose is not right for you then use a chair back or window ledge to rest the hands on as you come forward.

1. Begin on all fours as for the Cat pose (page 28), but have the toes turned under (A). Take a few breaths, feeling that the palms are firmly planted on the floor.

2. On an exhalation, take the buttocks back to the heels (B).

3. Breathe in, and on the next out breath let the knees float up off the floor, taking the buttocks back and up, while the arms straighten. Don't rush to straighten the knees or get the heels down to the floor.

4. Breathe freely and feel the spine elongate, taking the tailbone up into the air (C). Push gently down with the heels of the hands to take the upper body back towards the legs, sending the weight through the legs. Be sure not to strain or force the body back.

A.

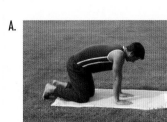

B.

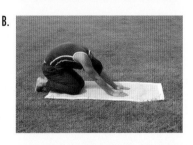

C.

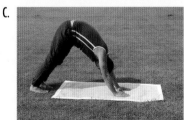

5. Keeping the balls of the feet on the floor, lift and lower each heel one at a time as if walking on the spot to create freedom in the hips, knees and ankles. If you are able to without creating tension or straining, take the heels to the ground to achieve the maximum stretch to the legs. Do not hold the posture for too long and remember to breathe freely throughout.

6. To come out, bend the arms and knees and come back to all fours. Then take the buttocks back and rest for a moment or two in the Swan or Child pose (page 36).

Ardha Sarvangasana or Half Shoulder Stand

Caution:
Not suitable for uncontrolled high blood pressure, heart, serious eye or ear problems or an enlarged thyroid. It is also not recommended while menstruating.

Benefits:
The thyroid gland is stimulated, there is improved blood flow to the brain and it relieves stress and headaches. Flexibility in the neck is improved.

1. Lie on your back in a straight line, with the palms alongside, or just under, the buttocks (A). In this posture the pressure is on the upper back, shoulders and back of the neck so you may want to have a blanket underneath you if your mat is on a hard floor.

2. Bend the knees and bring them up towards the stomach. As you exhale, press down with the arms and lift the hips from the floor (B). Place the palms of the hands on each side of the pelvis to support it (C). The upper body should be at an angle to the floor as shown. Slowly straighten the legs diagonally over the body. Breathe freely and hold the pose for a few breaths.

3. Carefully come out of the posture by reversing these steps. The neck should feel relaxed throughout. If you notice any pressure in the throat, neck or face then slowly come out of the posture.

A.

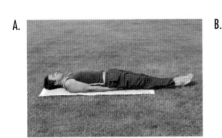

B.

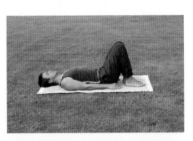

C.

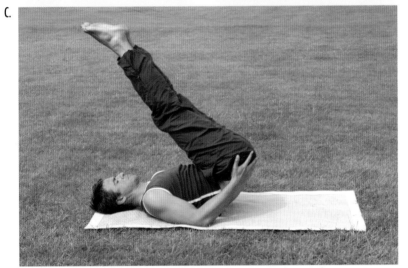

Sarvangasana or Shoulder Stand

Caution:
As for Half Shoulder Stand (page 86).
Benefits:
As for Half Shoulder Stand but more pronounced.
Modification:
Sit against a wall, sideways on and with the legs
out in front of you. Lift the buttock closest to the
wall so that it rests on the skirting. Lean back on
the hands and at the same time swivel the body
round so that both buttocks are against
the wall and the legs straight up the wall.

1. Lie on the floor as for the Half Shoulder Stand (A) and come up into the Ardha Sarvangasana for a breath or two (B).

2. Without forcing the movement, straighten the back and move the hands further up the back towards the shoulderblades (avoid pressing on the spine). Do this gradually and give the body time to adjust and open up.

3. In the full posture the whole body is perpendicular to the floor with the upper arms and hands providing support (C).

4. To come down, bend the knees towards the chest and slowly lower the body to the floor.

A.

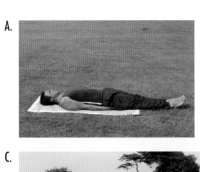

B.

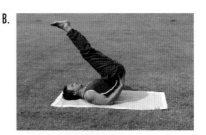

C.

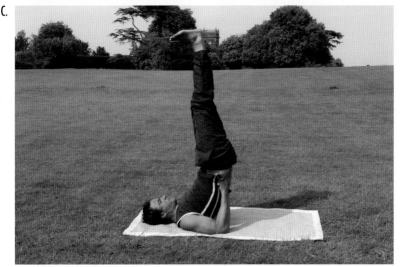

Halasana or Plough Pose

Caution:

As for Half Shoulder Stand on page 86. You should not practice Halasana if you have a slipped disc, hernia or a serious back problem, for example, arthritis of the neck.

Benefits:

All the internal organs are massaged, bringing about improved function. The abdominal muscles are strengthened and the spinal nerves are toned.

Modification:

If your feet don't reach the ground behind you, then rest them on a chair (B).

1. From shoulder stand (page 88) take the legs over the head so that the feet rest on the floor behind you. The hands should continue to support the back as the legs straighten and you relax into the posture. Ideally the back is perpendicular to the floor (A).

2. Hold the pose, breathing freely for a minute or two; later you can build up to holding the posture for five minutes.

3. Come out of the posture by bringing the legs up off the floor and then bending them and coming down as for Sarvangasana.

A.

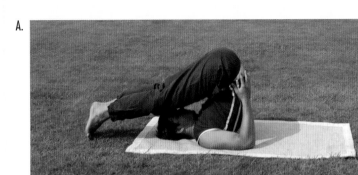

B.

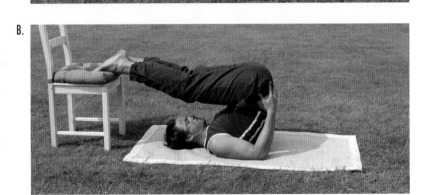

91

Jathara Parivartanasana or Lying Twist

Caution:

It is safer for the back, to raise and lower the legs bent rather than straight. Keep the head in the central position if you have neck problems, or if you find that turning the head makes the shoulder lift off the floor. This is the full posture but the modification may be more suitable for beginners.

Benefits:

Twisting strengthens the muscles supporting the spine and encourages flexibility in the spine. The abdominal organs are massaged and strengthened. Regular practice has a slimming and firming effect to the waist, tummy, hips and buttocks. It is said to be good for lifting low spirits or depression.

Modification:

Supine limber 6 (page 18–19) is a modification of Jathara Parivartanasana. This version can also be done with the legs together, as if they are glued along the inner sides.

1. Lie on the floor in a straight line then take the arms out to shoulder height, palms up or down (A).

2. Bend and lift the left leg (B) with an exhalation, then straighten it as you inhale.

3. From that position, as you breathe out, lower the leg over to the right side of the body, ensuring that both shoulder blades retain contact with the floor (C). If the foot doesn't touch the floor when out to the opposite side, then rest it on a block or cushion.

4. Breathe in, and on the out breath turn the head to face the left (D).

5. Close the eyes, breathe freely and try to feel the spine and shoulders releasing as you exhale. Come back to the starting position carefully and with awareness.

A.

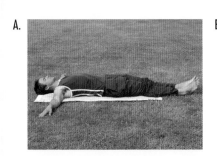

B.

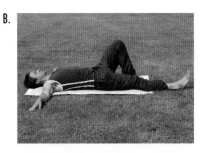

C.

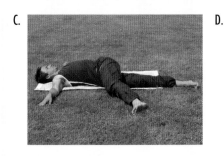

D.

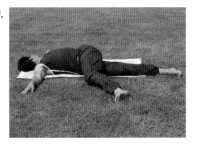

Ardha Matsyendrasana or Half Spinal Twist

Caution:
Those with a slipped disc or sciatica should take great care when practising this posture.

Benefits:
Similar to Jathara Parivartanasana.

Modifications:
Once you have crossed the right leg over the left, bend the left leg and bring the foot alongside the right buttock, and vice versa for the other side.

A more advanced version is to wrap the back arm around the back of the waist, but only do this if you feel strong and steady in the pose (E).

1. Sit with the legs straight out in front of you. Bend the right leg and place the foot on the floor beside the outer edge of the left leg, toes facing forwards (A).

2. Turning the torso towards the right, place the left arm along the outer edge of the right thigh (B). Take a breath or two in this position.

3. Lift the right arm and draw a circle with it behind you, pushing gently with the left arm against the right thigh (C).

4. Turn the head slowly around to the right as your gaze follows the hand, then place the fingertips on the floor behind you. You should now be looking over the right shoulder (D). Try not to lean on the back hand — you may need to have a block or a book to rest the back hand on if this helps to keep the spine straight and perpendicular to the floor.

A.

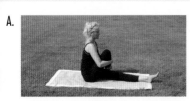

B.

C.

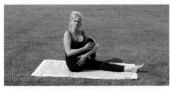

D.

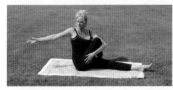

E.

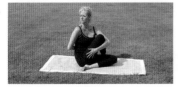

5. Close the eyes and breathe freely, focusing on relaxing into the posture with the exhalation. Hold for a minute or two, before slowly bringing the back hand and torso around to the front. Release the legs and give them a rub before practising on the other side.

Modified Twist

Sit sideways on a straight-back chair with the right side of the body next to the chair back and feet on the floor. Make sure the spine is straight.

On an exhalation, slowly turn the body towards the right, take the hands around with you and hold the chair back. Keep your feet on the floor. Those without neck problems can then turn the head to look over the right shoulder. Hold the pose, breathing freely for 20–30 seconds. Slowly turn to face the front again on an out breath, then switch sides and repeat the twist.

Surya Namaskar or Salute to the Sun

Surya means sun and Namaskara means salutations. In ancient times the sun was worshipped every day as it symbolises spiritual consciousness.
Surya Namaskar is a series of twelve postures, which, once learnt, should flow smoothly from one to the other.

Caution:

Surya Namaskar is vigorous, and it is not recommended that it is used by the beginner to commence a yoga session. It should not be practised if you have uncontrolled high blood pressure, heart problems or have had a stroke. Those with back problems should be careful too.

Benefits:

Stimulates and balances the respiratory, circulatory and digestive systems. Tones the whole body. Brings about a feeling of wellbeing.

1. Stand at the front of your mat in Tadasana with the hands in Namaste at the heart centre (A).

2. Breathe in and stretch up and back. If you have back problems bend the knees when you do this (B).

3. On an out breath, bend the body forward from the hips and come into Utthanasana, placing the palms down and the fingertips in line with the tips of the toes (C).

4. Step back with the right foot, keeping the toes tucked under and drop the right knee to the floor. The chest moves forward while you look up (D).

5. Step the left foot back in line with the right and come up into Adho Mukha Svanasana (E).

6. Lower the knees, chest and chin to the floor (F). Ideally they should all touch the floor at the same time.

A.
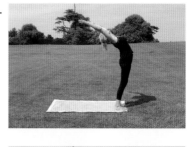

B.

C.
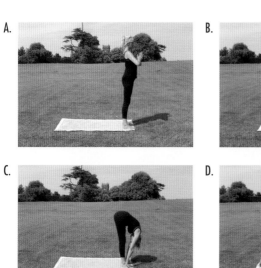

D.
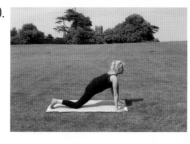

E.
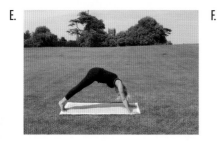

F.
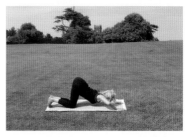

Surya Namaskar or Salute to the Sun (continued)

7. Push the upper body forwards between the hands and come into Bhujangasana although the arms can remain slightly bent (G).

8. Push into the floor with the hands, taking the buttocks up and back and come into Adho Mukha Svanasana again (H).

9. Step forwards with the right foot, placing the toe tips in line with the fingertips if possible, dropping the left knee to the floor and bringing the chest forwards and looking up (I).

10. Step the left foot forwards so the toe and fingertips line up and the forehead is close to the legs (Utthanasana) (J).

11. Breathe in and come out of Utthanasana, taking the arms up and back as in step 2 (K).

12. Bring the hands to Namaste and lower them down to the heart centre. Take a couple of recovery breaths in Tadasana (L).

This completes half a round. For the second half, you lead with the left foot in Steps 4 and 9.

Note

Beginners should start by practising one or two rounds and then gradually build up with one extra round every few weeks, if desired. Generally, two or three rounds are practised in a typical yoga class.

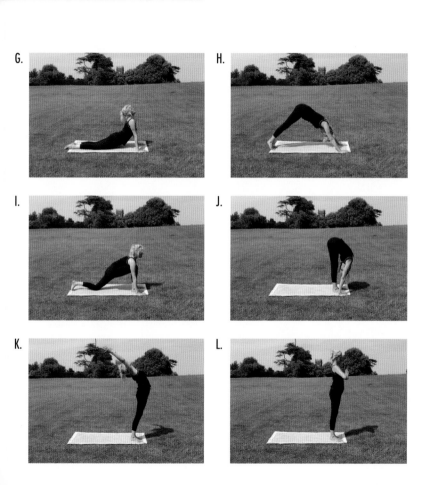

G.

H.

I.

J.

K.

L.

99

Home Practice

Yoga is ideally suited to practising in the home, in the garden or even on a beach. Remember to limber up well before practising the asanas and try to take the spine in all directions. It is good to start the session (especially after a busy day) lying in semi-supine, focusing on the breath, allowing yourself to unwind. If you only have 10-15 minutes then spend a few moments limbering up and then concentrate on practising one or two postures, perhaps twice each. Follow with pranayama and/or relaxation. Alternatively, use these suggested sequences.

Sequence 1

(about thirty minutes)

Spend five to six minutes limbering up, e.g. Apanasana, gentle lying twist, stretching through with the breath, neck and shoulder limbers and foot and leg limbers.

Butterfly followed by Baddha Konasana (page 38)
Tadasana (page 42)
Trikonasana (page 48)
Rag Doll (page 58)
Vrksasana (page 60)
Sphinx (page 66)
Ardha Salabhasana (page 71)
Swan (page 36)
Adho Mukha Svanasana (page 84)
Child (page 36)
Ardha Matsyendrasana (page 94)
Paschimottanasana (page 78)
Relaxation (five to ten minutes)

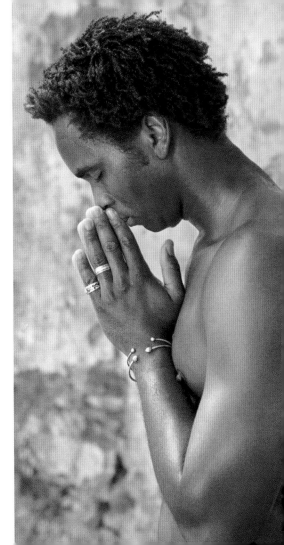

Sequence 2

(about thirty minutes)

Four to five minutes limbering up, e.g. stretching through with the breath, knee circling, cycling, pelvic lifting, hamstring stretch and gentle lying twist.

Sequence Three

(about forty minutes)

Spend eight to ten minutes limbering up,
e.g. stretching through with the breath, Apanasana,
hamstring stretch, pelvic lifting, knee circling and
neck and shoulder limbers.

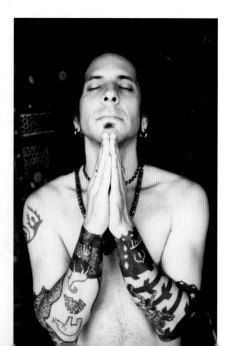

Dandasana for the legs and feet
limbers (pages 37, 26)

Baddha Konasana (page 38)

Gomukhasana (page 40)

Trikonasana (page 48)

Parsvakonsasana (page 54)

Rag Doll (page 58)

Tadasana (page 42)

Garudasana (page 64)

Majariasana (page 28)

Adho Mukha Svanasana (page 84)

Bhujangasana (page 68)

Salabhasana (page 70)

Swan or Child (page 36)

Jathara Parivartanasana (page 92)

Ardha Sarvangasana (page 86)

Hug and rock (page 74)

Upavista Konasana (page 82)

Pranayama (pages 120–125

Relaxation (five to ten minutes)

The DVD accompanying this book includes
a yoga session lasting approximately one hour.
If you prefer not to use the DVD then follow the
list of positions below for the same routine.

Relaxation

Relaxing at the end of a yoga session is very important as it gives the body and mind time to become still and absorb the benefits of the asanas. The more you practice relaxation the more you will be able to use it throughout the day.

Try to spend at least ten minutes relaxing after your yoga practice, although if you only have 10-15 minutes in which to practice, try to allow three to five minutes for relaxation.

Try not to let thoughts which pop into the mind take over – simply acknowledge the thought and then let it float away on an out breath.

Preparation

The body can become cool during relaxation so ensure that you have a blanket and/or some warm clothing to put on. For added comfort you may like to have a blanket under the body, too. Try to ensure that you will not be disturbed during your relaxation.

Lie in Savasana (page 20) checking that the body is straight, the back of the neck long, the feet at least hip width apart and flopping out to the sides, and the arms a little distance from the sides of the body, with the palms uppermost and the fingers curling naturally. Close the eyes. If you need more support for the lower back, lie in semi-supine.

If the back of the head does not touch the ground without tilting the chin up towards the ceiling, thereby shortening the back of the neck, then rest the head on a block or folded towel to keep the back of the neck long.

Alternatively, if you are unable to lie on the floor or feel that you will fall asleep, sit in a position where you know you will be comfortable for the duration of the relaxation. Whether sitting on the floor or in a straight-back chair, make sure that the spine is straight.

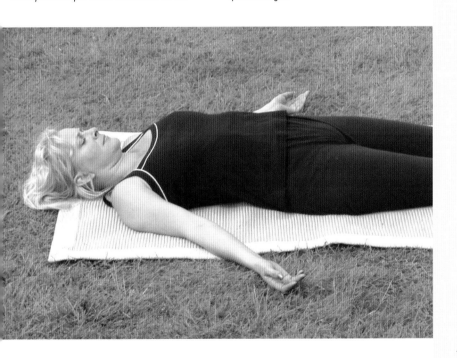

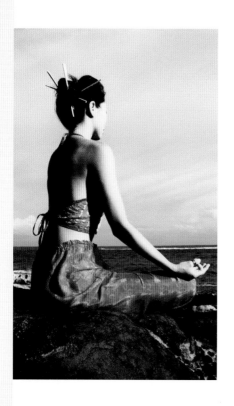

Relaxation 1

Send your mind's eye around the body checking for areas of tension. If you need to make any adjustments to the position of the body then do so now.

Become aware of the breath, don't try to change it, just follow its movement. The breath may be long and deep or short and shallow, or anywhere in between — just accept how it is at the moment.

Take the attention to the feet and turn the toes under, really tensing the muscles in the feet, then slowly let go of the tension.

Now tense the whole of both legs and then gradually release. Feel that the legs and feet are sinking softly into the ground.

Now take the awareness to the hands and make fists with them, then slowly release. Next, stretch through to the fingertips, stretching the muscles in the arms, hands and upper body. Then slowly let go. Feel that the upper body, arms and legs are sinking into the floor beneath you.

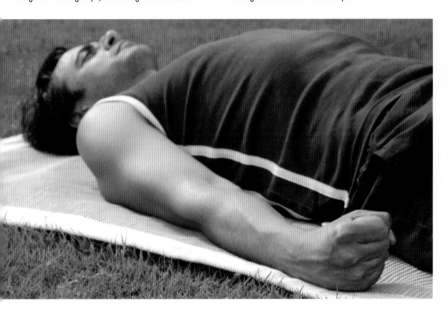

Next, gently tighten the abdominal muscles and clench the buttocks, before slowly letting go of the tension. Feel that the lower body is sinking down.

Finally, screw up the face in an exaggerated scowl and then gradually release the muscles and feel the head sink down into the ground. Feel that the body relaxes more with every out breath. Allow yourself to be still and peaceful for a few moments more.

To come out of relaxation, slowly start to wriggle the fingers and toes. Then gently roll the head from side to side before bringing it back to the central position. Now, either enjoy a gentle stretch through the whole body, taking the arms overhead on the in breath and releasing them back to the sides as you exhale, or draw the knees in towards the chest and gently rock from side to side.

With the legs bent, roll over to the right side and open the eyes, then slowly push up to a sitting position.

Relaxation 2

Once in Savasana (or any other comfortable position) become aware of the breath. Don't try to change it, just be aware of what it is doing. The breath may be long and deep or short and shallow, or anywhere in between — just accept how it is at the moment. Concentrating on the breath calms the mind and quietens the body, slowing the pulse rate and lowering the blood pressure.

Now take two or three deeper breaths, and see if you can make the exhalation longer than the inhalation. Try to feel that you are letting go as you breathe in this way.

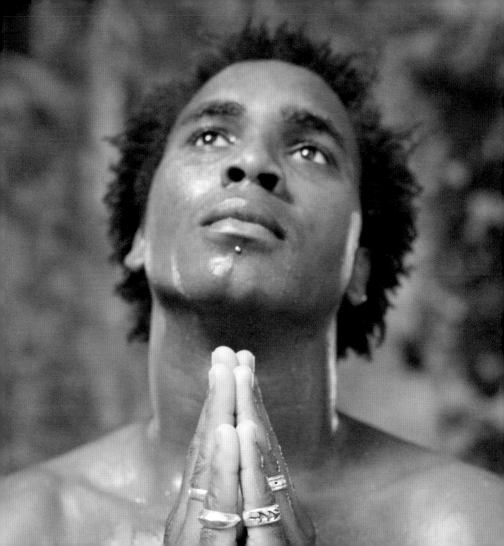

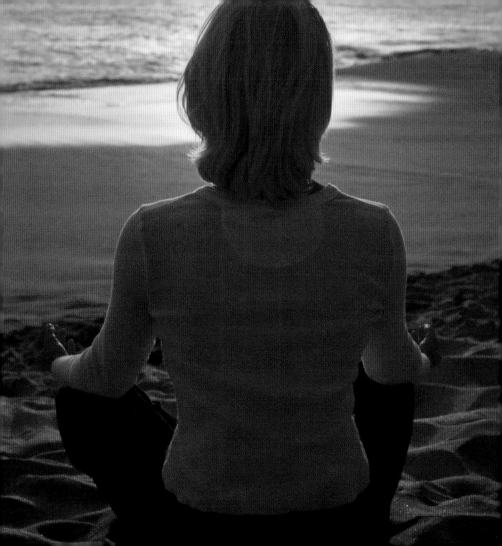

Now bring the awareness to the parts of the body which come into contact with the floor.

Feel the:
- back of the head on the floor (pause);
- shoulder blades on the floor (pause);
- arms and hands on the floor (pause);
- spine on the floor (pause);
- buttocks on the floor (pause);
- backs of the legs on the floor (pause);
- heels on the floor (pause),

feel each part of your body becoming heavier as you relax. Know that your body is well supported by the ground and let yourself bathe in the sea of tranquillity around, and within, you.

To come out of this relaxation, slowly start to wriggle the fingers and toes. Then gently roll the head from side to side before bringing it back to the central position. Gently stretch the entire body, or draw the knees in towards the chest and gently rock from side to side.

Bend the legs, roll over to the right side before opening your eyes, then gently push yourself up into a sitting position.

Note

It may be worth recording these relaxation techniques so that you can listen to them, rather than trying to memorise them.

Relaxation can also be practised while listening to some peaceful music or the sounds of nature, such as the sea lapping on the seashore.

Expanding the Life Force

Pranayama in its simplest terms is control of the breath but it is actually much more than that. Prana is defined as 'life force' and 'ayama' means extension or expansion.

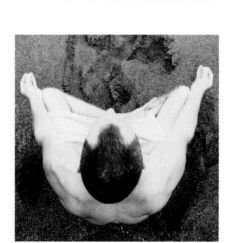

Pranayama can be thought of as the means of expanding the life force within us. It establishes regular breathing patterns and helps to clear physical, emotional and mental blocks which can lead to ill-health.

Patanjali defines Pranayama in his Yoga Sutras:
"Pranayama is the conscious, deliberate regulation of the breath replacing unconscious patterns of breathing. It is possible only after a reasonable mastery of asana practice." Chapter 2, Sutra 49.

Humans breathe approximately 21,600 times a day, or fifteen times per minute. The ancient 'rishis' (seers or sages) observed that animals with a slow breath rate, such as tortoises, lived longer than animals with a fast breath rate, such as birds. From this observation they recognised the value of slow breathing for longevity.

Deep breathing massages the heart and internal organs; it encourages healthy venous return and good lymph drainage. The lungs are used more fully and this, in turn, allows for improved intake of oxygen and better exchange at the cellular level.

The spine moves more with deeper breaths and this helps to keep it healthy. Breathing deeply while practising asanas allows release and opening.

Pranayama helps to still the mind and bring about a sense of calmness and wellbeing which can lead to improved concentration.

"When the body is in silent stillness, breathe rhythmically through the nostrils with a peaceful ebbing and flowing of breath. The chariot of the mind is drawn by wild horses, and those wild horses have to be tamed." Svetasvatara Upanishad, Part 2.

Prana flows through the body along 'nadis', which are known as the meridians in the Chinese system. It is believed that there are 72,000 nadis or channels in the body.

The three main nadis are:

'Sushumna' nadi which runs along the spinal column, is the channel for nervous energy and awakening spiritual consciousness. 'Ida' and 'Pingala' nadis, cross over the spinal column at the points of the chakras as shown overleaf. Ida nadi passes the left nostril, conveys lunar energy and controls the mental processes. Pingala, which crosses the right nostril, conveys solar energy and controls the vital processes.

Prana must flow freely through the nadis as any blockage can cause illness. Asana and Pranayama practices help to keep the nadis open.

Energy Centres

The word Chakra is literally translated from Sanskrit as wheel or circle, but they are energy centres. There are seven main chakras in the body

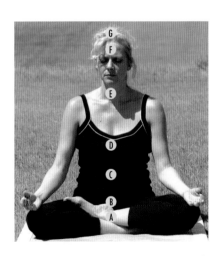

Mooladhara (A) or Base Chakra is situated at the base of the spine, just above the anus. It influences elimination from the body and is linked to the earth and our sense of smell. Represented by a red, four-petalled lotus flower, it is the source of all energy in mankind and the universe. This energy is represented by a coiled snake known as Kundalini which lays dormant in Mooladhara until awakened through yogic practices.

Swadhistana (B) or Support of Life Breath Centre is situated in the genital area and is linked with water and our sense of taste. It is represented by an orange, six-petalled lotus.

Manipura (C) or Jewel City Centre is situated in the solar plexus area and is linked to fire and sight. It influences the digestive system and is represented by a yellow, ten-petalled lotus.

Anahata (D) or Unstruck Sound Centre is located at the centre of the chest and is also known as the heart centre. It is the centre of unconditional love and physically is associated with the heart and lungs. It is represented by a green, 12-petalled lotus.

Vishuddhi (E) or Great Purity Centre is located in the throat. It influences the thyroid and parathyroid glands and is linked with sound, expression and creativity. It is represented by a blue, 16-petalled lotus.

Ajna (F) or Command Centre is situated in the middle of the forehead and is also known as the 'third eye.' This is where wisdom and intuition develop. It is represented by an indigo, two-petalled lotus and it is here that ida and pingala converge with sushumna.

Sahasrara (G) or 1000 Petalled Lotus Centre is located on the crown of the head. It is the centre of self-realisation.

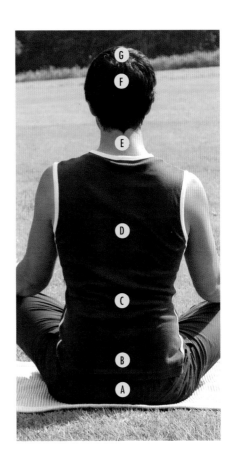

Seated Positions

The seated positions are used to practise Pranayama (yogic breathing techniques) and meditation. The purpose of practising yogic asanas is to prepare the body for long periods of meditation in a seated position

It is not necessary to get into the full lotus (Padmasana) as there are many achievable alternative sitting positions and remember, a straight-backed chair can be used if you are not able to sit on the floor.

In all cross-legged sitting positions, remember to alternate the legs so that you don't become accustomed to having a particular foot closest to the body every time.

Always come out of the pose if you are experiencing discomfort. Take care when coming out of cross-legged poses to avoid injury to the knees and rub the legs or roll them gently from side to side to ease them out.

1. Sukhasana or Easy Pose

Sit on the floor with the legs crossed at the ankles. Try to have the knees as low as possible, but do not push them down to the ground. Keep the spine straight, the back of the neck long and the chin parallel with the floor. The hands should be resting softly on each thigh but do not stretch the arms so that the hands reach the knees – try to have the upper arms close to the sides of the body (A).

Often it is useful to sit on a yoga block or a folded blanket as this will allow the pelvis to tilt and the knees to lower more towards the ground. You may

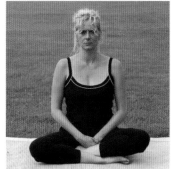

A.

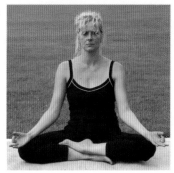

B.

find that you need to have a couple of blocks to be comfortable. It can be difficult keeping the spine straight and you may find it helpful to sit with the back against a wall to prevent you slumping.

2. *Siddhasana or Perfect Pose*

Sit with the legs straight out in front of you, then bend the right leg and place the heel against the perineum (the area between the genitals and anus) with the sole of the foot flat against the inside of the left thigh. Now bend the left leg and place the left foot on top of the right. If having the feet like this is uncomfortable, place a folded cloth over the right foot to act as a cushion between the feet. The knees should ideally be on the ground. Now slip the left toes into the space between the calf and thigh of the right leg. Remember that the spine needs to be straight (B).

3. Ardha Padmasana or Half Lotus Pose

Sit with the legs straight out in front of you and then bend one leg, placing the sole of the foot along the inner thigh of the other leg, with the heel close to the perineum. Now bend the other leg and place the foot on top of the other thigh, as close as is comfortable to the abdomen. As with the other sitting postures, the spine needs to be straight and the body upright (C).

4. Padmasana or Lotus Pose

Do not attempt this posture until you have strengthened the legs and have achieved good flexibility of the knees. It should not be practised by anyone with weak or injured knees.

Sit with the legs straight out in front of you and then carefully bend one leg and place the foot on top of the opposite thigh, with the sole of the foot facing up (D). Then bend the other leg and place the foot on top of the other thigh.

Both knees should touch the ground. The hands should rest in the lap one on top of the other (E) or in Chin or Jnana Mudra (F), where the first finger is folded so that the tip rests at the base of the thumb and the other three fingers are straight. In Chin Mudra the palms are facing upwards and in Jnana Mudra they are touching the legs.

C.

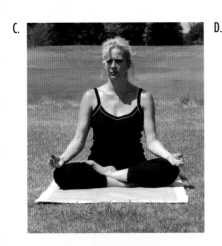

D.

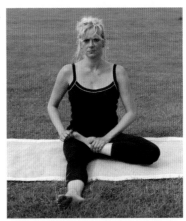

E.

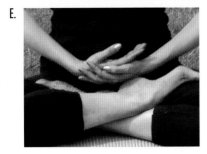

F.

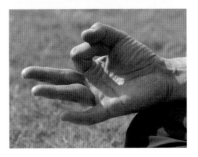

The Pranayama Practices

Caution:

Pranayama practices can have powerful effects physically and emotionally and it is always best to learn these practices under the guidance of a qualified yoga teacher. If you become dizzy or feel strain in the head or eyes, stop the practice immediately and let the breath return to normal. If you start to feel over-emotional then you should also stop straight away. People with uncontrolled high blood pressure, or heart, serious eye or ear problems should never retain the breath (this book does not give information about breath retention).

Benefits (Full Yogic Breath):

Stress, anxiety or fear causes a primitive reflex that results in a chemical reaction in the body to prepare it for 'fight or flight'. As a result, the breath quickens so that only the upper chest is used. Full yogic breathing is useful at any time in calming the nerves in stressful situations.

Many of us draw the abdomen in when we breathe in but this is actually the reverse of the natural process. Don't become worried and tense if you discover that you are breathing in this way, however. Naturally the abdomen and chest area expand on the in breath and relax back on the out breath. Try to relax and encourage the natural process to happen.

Preparation

Try to practice at the same time every day: early morning or in the evening are generally considered to be best. In a yoga class, Pranayama is generally practised after the asanas and before relaxation.

Find a quiet, comfortable space to practice – one where you are unlikely to be disturbed. Do not practice immediately after eating: allow a couple of hours after a heavy meal. On the other hand, do not try to practice if you are hungry.

Traditionally, Pranayama is practised properly in a seated position. Remember that the spine moves with the breath, so it is important to keep the spine straight throughout the practice.

Full Yogic Breath

There are three stages to the full yogic breath and it is important that you learn each one before trying the full practice. Take your time to do this.

1. Abdominal (Diaphragmatic) Breathing

It is good to learn this while in a seated pose or lying in Savasana (or semi-supine). Rest your hands gently on the abdomen with the fingers pointing to the centre and the thumbs just along the lower edge of the ribs (A).

Try to become aware that the abdomen rises as you breathe in, causing the fingers to move slightly away from each other. Don't force the abdomen to rise up as this will create tension.

Sense that it is the abdomen only which is expanding and feel that the rib cage is passive. Continue breathing in this way for two or three minutes.

A.
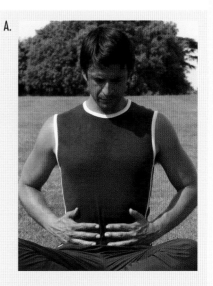

2. Thoracic Breathing

Thoracic breathing can also be learned while lying in Savasana. For this method of breathing move the hands further up to the sides of the chest (A).

Spend a moment or two observing the breath and then send the awareness to the ribs and as you inhale feel the rib cage expand. Again, don't force the rib cage to expand. On the exhalation, feel the rib cage contract. Continue breathing in this way for two or three minutes.

3. Clavicular Breathing

Clavicular breathing can be practised lying down or in a seated position. The hands should be resting on the chest with the fingertips touching the clavicles (B).

Spend a few moments watching the breath before inhaling and sensing the upper part of the lungs expanding and the ribs opening up, causing the collar bones to move up slightly. On the out breath feel the ribs contract and the collar bones drop. Continue breathing in this way for two to three minutes.

A.

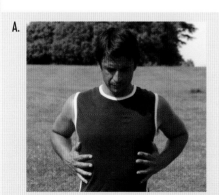

B.

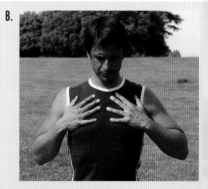

4. Full Yogic Breath

Once you are confident in the three stages described earlier, you can bring it all together for the full practice. Assume a comfortable position, either lying with the arms resting on the floor or sitting with the spine straight and the hands in the lap or resting on each thigh.

Breathe in slowly and first sense the abdomen rise, then the chest expand outwards and upwards until the ribs are fully expanded, and lastly feel the collar bones move up slightly. This breath should be one flowing movement without strain or jerks.
Be aware of the natural pause that exists between the end of the in breath and the start of the out breath, but don't hold your breath deliberately.

Breathe out slowly in the same flowing manner, sensing the collar bones and upper chest contracting, then the remainder of the rib cage and, finally, feel the abdomen drop down. You can very

gently tighten the abdominal muscles down towards the end of the out breath to expel a little more air so long as you do not strain or create tension.

Be aware of the natural pause that exists between the end of the out breath and the start of the in breath, but again, don't hold the breath out deliberately.

This completes one round of the yogic breath. Practice up to five rounds to begin with and then build up slowly to about ten minutes a day.

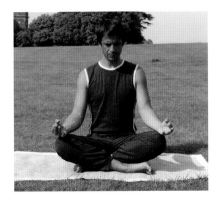

Nadi Sodhana or Alternate Nostril Breathing

In this practice we breathe in through the left nostril, exhale through the right nostril, then inhale through the right nostril and breathe out through the left nostril. This is one round of alternate nostril breathing.

Benefits:

Alternate nostril breathing is calming and can help if you have a headache or suffer from insomnia.

During the practice the carbon dioxide is expelled more efficiently and the whole body receives an extra supply of oxygen. It clears blockages in the Nadis and balances Ida and Pingala, allowing Sushumna nadi to flow, and this leads to spiritual awakening.

Modification:

If at first you find it difficult to concentrate on breathing through alternate nostrils, block off the right nostril and take three or five breaths in and out through the left nostril. Follow this by blocking off the left nostril and taking the same number of breaths through the right nostril. If the right arm becomes tired, lower it and imagine that you are breathing in and out through alternate nostrils.

1. The right hand is used to block off each nostril in turn. Bring the hand up to the face and rest the first and middle fingers on the forehead between the eyebrows. Rest the thumb on the right side of the nose just on the bony part above the nostrils and the ring finger on the left. The little finger can be straight or folded in. Try to have the elbow pointing straight down and not out at an angle as this may cause tension in the shoulder.

A.

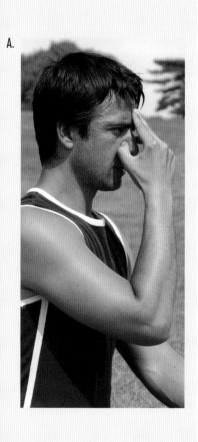

2. If you want to close the eyes, then take a couple of breaths in and out through the nose with the right hand in position but not blocking off the nostrils.

3. Press gently against the right nostril with the thumb to close off that nostril and breathe in through the left nostril (A). At the end of the inhalation, place the ring finger against the left nostril to stop air escaping. Now release the pressure of the thumb from the right nostril and exhale.

4. With the left nostril still closed off, inhale through the right nostril and close it off with the thumb at the end of the in breath. Release the ring finger from the left nostril and breathe out through the left. This completes one round. To begin with, practice three to five rounds and then gradually increase the rounds to last about two or three minutes.

Achieving Oneness

Many people think of meditation as a religious practice, but it is actually a spiritual practice, not requiring belief in any particular god or deity.

The ultimate goal of meditation is oneness with the higher self, the universe, God, reality – whichever name you prefer to think of it by.

To meditate one needs to be in a quiet, comfortable place away from distractions for ten to fifteen minutes to begin with. Try to practice at the same time every day. Do not practice immediately after eating: try to allow a couple of hours after a heavy meal.

Caution:

As meditation involves looking within, it is generally not recommended for people who are depressed or for those with epilepsy, except under the guidance of an experienced teacher.

Jyoti Meditation

This is a meditation on the universal light and is known as the Jyoti Meditation. You will need a candle for this meditation.

Sit in one of the seated postures (pages 116-118) with the spine straight (sit with the back against a wall for support if necessary). If using an upright chair, ensure that the back is straight and the feet are flat on the floor.

Gently focus the gaze on the candle flame. Breathe freely while you watch the flame change shape, colour, size etc. Now close your eyes and try to see the flame behind your closed eyelids. Feel that the

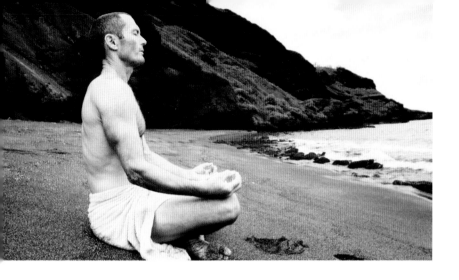

light from the flame is being drawn into your heart, which opens up like a lotus flower, petal by petal.

The light is now growing and slowly filling every cell of your body. First you were in the light, then the light was in you. Now you are the light. The light continues to grow, filling the room and beyond. On and on it grows as the light within you merges with the light in all other beings. Spend a few moments feeling yourself and the world being healed and strengthened by the light.

Very gradually, the light becomes smaller. Eventually it is the size of a candle flame again. Let this small light rest in your heart, so it is always there to call on if you need to.

Slowly start bringing the awareness back to the outside – be aware of your breath. Become aware of the contact points between your body and the floor. Gently wriggle the fingers and toes. When you feel ready to, open your eyes and enjoy a stretch through.

127

Enhancing your Life

Yoga is suitable for most people and can be used solely for the physical benefits or taken to greater depths, which lead to a spiritual path.

In the classical yoga text *Hatha Yoga Pradipika*, Swatmarama said:

"Asanas are the starting point as they form the first stage of Hatha Yoga. Asanas make one firm, free from diseases, and light of limb."
Chapter 1, V 17.

We may not become completely 'free from diseases' through our yoga practice, but there is no doubt that the body will become strengthened, toned and more supple. Our posture and respiration will improve and this all leads to a healthier body.

Practising yoga with awareness will calm the mind and improve concentration. We are more able to control the emotions, achieving greater relaxation of mind and body. Whatever the level at which you choose to practice your yoga, it will enhance your life.

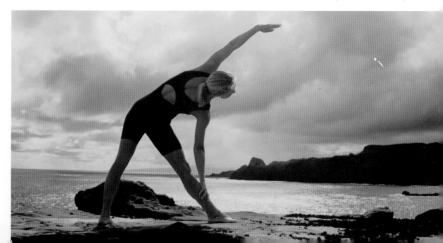